weight
control
THROUGH DIET & EXERCISE

Dr Geoffrey Webb

TEACH YOURSELF BOOKS

For UK orders: please contact Bookpoint Ltd, 39 Milton Park, Abingdon, Oxon OX14 4TD. Telephone: (44) 01235 400414, Fax: (44) 01235 400454. Lines are open from 9.00 - 6.00, Monday to Saturday, with a 24 hour message answering service. Email address: orders@bookpoint.co.uk

For U.S.A. order enquiries: please contact McGraw-Hill Customer Services, P.O. Box 545, Blacklick, OH 43004-0545, U.S.A. Telephone: 1-800-722-4726. Fax: 1-614-755-5645.

Long renowned as the authoritative source for self-guided learning – with more than 30 million copies sold worldwide – the *Teach Yourself* series includes over 200 titles in the fields of languages, crafts, hobbies, sports, and other leisure activities.

A catalogue entry for this title is available from The British Library.

Library of Congress Catalog Card Number: On file

First published in UK 1998 by Hodder Headline Plc, 338 Euston Road, London, NW1 3BH.

First published in US 1998 by Contemporary Books, A Division of The McGraw-Hill Companies, 1 Prudential Plaza, 130 East Randolph Street, Chicago, Illinois 60601 U.S.A.

The 'Teach Yourself' name and logo are registered trade marks of Hodder & Stoughton Ltd.

Typeset by Transet Limited, Coventry, England.
Printed in Great Britain for Hodder & Stoughton Educational, a division of Hodder Headline Plc, 338 Euston Road, London NW1 3BH by Cox & Wyman Ltd, Reading, Berkshire.

Impression number   10 9 8 7 6 5
Year   2002

CONTENTS

PREFACE

Hundreds of diet books have been published in the last few years, so why have I written yet another? This book is about dieting and weight control, but is not intended to be yet another addition to the endless list of diet books. In the spirit of the much-respected *Teach Yourself* series, I have tried to write something that will improve knowledge and understanding of weight control and the reasons for excess weight gain as well as providing readers with advice about practical measures to help in controlling their weight.

I see the main audience for this book as the very large number of adults who, whilst not seriously obese, are concerned about their current weight or concerned to prevent excessive weight gain as they move towards middle-age and beyond. The book is also aimed at all those parents who are interested in guiding the lifestyle and diet of their children in ways that will reduce the chances of them becoming victim to the epidemic of obesity that is currently sweeping through the industrialised world. I do not believe that this book alone is likely to solve the problems of those people with severe obesity that has resisted many previous weight loss attempts. Although the general strategies suggested in this book are appropriate for treating severe and persistent obesity, these people will probably need professional help in designing an appropriate weight loss programme and more especially in providing support, encouragement and coping strategies to help them stick to this programme over the many months that they will need to follow it. In some cases, more aggressive treatments for their obesity may be considered justified, for example, very low calorie diets, anti-obesity drugs or even surgical treatments.

In Chapter 2, I have given a list of people for whom dieting and weight loss might be inappropriate unless under medical advice and supervision. I would in no way advocate that parents put their children on to reducing diets or even try to impose rigid low fat, low sugar, high fibre diets on them without such supervision. This may limit growth and development and may foster an unhealthy preoccupation with dieting and body shape that could encourage more children to develop eating disorders such as anorexia and bulimia. Although childhood obesity is increasing rather alarmingly it is still the exception rather than the rule. I am convinced that this rise in childhood obesity is, in any case, largely due to inactivity rather than a fatty or sugary diet.

When I started to write this book, I set myself a series of aims which are briefly mentioned below in the hope that they may help readers to understand the purpose of what is written and encourage them to persist with those sections which they may find difficult.

After reading Chapters 1 and 2, readers should be able to decide whether they are overweight, be able to gauge the severity of their weight problem and its likely impact upon the prospects for their future health and wellbeing. They should have a broad appreciation of the general dietary and lifestyle patterns that are conducive to better weight control and better health prospects generally, as well as some idea of how many calories they need and how much food this represents. They should have some appreciation of the scale of the problem of excessive weight gain, the alarmingly high rate of increase and thus why excessive fatness is a problem that needs to be considered a public health priority.

In Chapters 3 and 4, I have summarised current scientific understanding of the physiological mechanisms that control food intake and body weight and suggested reasons why these mechanisms appear to fail in so many people. In other words, I have tried to identify some of the reasons why we get fat. These chapters may prove challenging for the lay reader, especially Chapter 3. The physiology of weight control is a complex and rapidly evolving topic that is hard enough for scientists to keep abreast of. However, I do think that a wider understanding of the reasons for excessive weight gain and of the rationale for current treatments and preventive measures are important goals. Individual and public health measures to control obesity are more likely to be effective if people understand the reasoning behind the advice they are given and, more importantly, if they can be convinced that such advice is soundly based and has evidential support.

In Chapter 5, I have studied some of the various diet and weight loss strategies that have appeared in popular books (and elsewhere) over the years. I have then suggested why I believe many of these strategies to be unsound, even though many might achieve some weight loss if followed diligently. Some criteria for judging weight loss programmes are offered at the end of the chapter.

Finally, in Chapters 6, 7 and 8 I have offered some practical advice for achieving weight loss and/or preventing weight gain; both for individual dieters and for the population as a whole, which should help to reduce obesity rates. I have identified increased activity and a reduced fat diet as the priorities for better weight control and, of course, deliberate calorie restriction for reasonably rapid weight loss. More exercise and a lower fat diet should improve health and wellbeing directly, over and above their effects upon body weight and shape and examples are given of ways in which activity levels can be increased and fat and calorie intake reduced. The use of drugs and surgery to treat obesity is very briefly reviewed, but detailed discussion of these is beyond the scope of a self-help book such as this one.

I offer readers no easy way of losing weight, no painless cure for obesity. Any claims for such easy solutions should be treated with extreme scepticism; dieting and weight loss are difficult, painful and slow processes. I do, however, suggest general lifestyle and eating patterns that should lessen the risks of weight gain, as well as offering practical ways of reducing fat and calorie intake and of increasing the body's calorie expenditure. It is bordering on platitude, but nonetheless true, that if calorie intake is less than calorie use then weight loss is inevitable.

Throughout the book, the author has provided guidance and advice on issues relating to weight control, but a professional should be consulted for the undertaking and suitability of treatment.

1 | INTRODUCTION

Scope of the chapter

In this introductory chapter, I will try to answer some of the following basic questions:

- What is normal body composition and how is it measured?
- How are obesity and overweight defined and how can I decide whether I am overweight or obese?
- How widespread is obesity and how is its prevalence increasing?
- Which people within our societies are most at risk of gaining excess weight?
- How many calories do I need?
- How much food does my calorie requirement represent?

Normal body composition

Table 1.1 gives typical body compositions for a 'reference' young man and woman which are based upon survey measurements of thousands of Americans; they should not be regarded as ideal values. In the reference man, fat makes up about 10.5 kg (15 per cent) of the body weight and all but 2 kg of this is storage fat. The remaining 2 kg of 'essential fat' is fat in the bone marrow, brain and vital organs of the body which is an essential part of their structure. The 8.5 kg of storage fat is a store of energy that would help this man to survive for some weeks without any food and perhaps for many months on restricted rations.

In the reference female, fat accounts for 15.4 kg (27 per cent) of the body weight – therefore women have almost twice the percentage of fat that men have. The extra fat in our typical woman, is classified as essential fat and is the fat found in the breasts and in the pelvic region that is necessary for successful reproduction. A minimum threshold amount of body fat is necessary for fertility and proper menstrual cycling in women, and very underweight women stop menstruating until their fat stores are replenished. As a consequence of her extra fat, the typical woman also has a lower proportion of muscle in her body than the typical man.

Table 1.1 Body composition of typical young American men and women

	Man	**Woman**
Height (m)	1.74	1.64
Weight (kg)	70	57
Body Mass Index	23.1	21.2
Fat (kg)	10.5	15.4
% body weight	15%	27%
Essential fat (kg)	2.1	6.8
% body weight	3%	12%
Storage fat	8.4	8.6
% body weight	12%	15%
Bone (kg)	10.5	6.8
% body weight	14.9%	12%
All lean (kg)	49	34.6
% body weight	70.1%	61%
Muscle	31.4	20.5
% body weight	44.8%	36%

NB: 1 metre = about 39 inches
1 kilogram = about 2.2 pounds

Source: Adapted from Behnke, A R and Wilmore, J H, 1974. *Evaluation and regulation of body build and composition*. Englewood Cliffs, NJ : Prentice Hall.

Am I overweight?

I am not fat, just heavy-boned

The term obese strictly denotes a substantial excess of body fat. However, it is very difficult to measure fat content directly in living people and so some measure of weight in relation to height is usually used to indicate a person's degree of fatness – a person who is heavy for their height is assumed to be fat. In adults of the same sex and height, then, weight is a reasonable predictor of the amount of body fat despite some variation in frame size and in the amount of muscle. It is also true that in most adults, a high proportion of any substantial long-term changes in weight will be due to changes in the amount of fat. Stability of body weight usually means that body fat content is also stable. A few exceptions to these generalisations are discussed below.

Very muscular people

Body builders and other very muscular people may be heavy for their height without being fat; their high body weight is due to higher than usual amounts of muscle. They may even gain weight despite losing fat because of increasing muscle weight. Some very muscular American football players have, in the past, been rejected for military service because they were heavy and so mistakenly classified as obese.

Oedema and dehydration

Oedema (swelling of tissues due to excess fluid) can cause increases in weight without changes in body fat. Oedema is a symptom of a number of illnesses or conditions such as heart failure, liver disease, renal failure, pregnancy and even malnutrition. In some cases of malnutrition (for example in developing world children or hospital patients), oedema can raise the body weight so much that it obscures the person's malnourished state.

Dehydration can have the opposite effect to oedema, that is, loss of body weight without any loss of fat. Profuse sweating will result in rapid short-term weight loss. For example, a marathon runner may lose up to 7 kg (14 lb) of sweat on a warm day and without regular drinks, dehydration may lead to collapse. Any weight losses due to dehydration will be restored when the person quenches their thirst. Some devices that claim to produce large and rapid weight losses simply cause sweating – this miraculous weight loss is just due to water loss and will be equally miraculously and rapidly regained! One may well lose a few pounds in the sauna but then immediately replace them in the café (or bar!) afterwards.

The elderly

As people become elderly, so the amount of muscle and bone in the body tends to fall and is replaced by fat. This change of body composition with age means that even if one's body weight remains fairly stable, then over the years the amount of fat may increase substantially. A group of elderly people will have a higher average body fat content than a group of young adults of the same height and weight. Inactivity is one cause of this age-related change in body composition, and so maintaining physical activity levels as one gets older should reduce these changes. This change in body composition may be partly reversible, and strength training results in measurable increases in muscle bulk even in people in their eighties and nineties.

Crash diets

People may lose substantial amounts of weight, (say, 7–8 lb or 3–4 kg), in the first week of a 'crash diet' but much of this weight loss would not be fat but be due to:

- losses of animal starch or **glycogen** from the liver and muscles (glycogen is the body's store of carbohydrate that can be used during the first few hours of fasting but even a well-fed body contains only about a pound (0.5 kg) of glycogen);
- loss of protein (lean tissue);
- loss of water associated with this glycogen and protein – each pound (0.5 kg) of body glycogen or protein is associated with three pounds (1.5 kg) of water and so each pound of glycogen or protein lost is accompanied by three pounds of water;
- a decrease in the weight of the gut contents.

This rate of weight loss cannot be sustained in the longer term. Much of this initial, large weight loss will be regained equally quickly once the severity of the diet is relaxed and the body's glycogen stores are replenished. Very rapid weight loss almost inevitably means undue loss of energy-burning muscle and lean tissue as well as fat.

Some height/weight measures

Weight-for-height tables

In the past, weight-for-height tables were the most common way of assessing people's weight status. These tables list the desirable weight ranges for men and women of any particular height and age. Three desirable ranges are given for each height and for each sex depending upon frame size, for example, whether the person is of light, medium or heavy build. A person is said to be obese if they are more than 20 per cent over their ideal weight range; and underweight if they are more than 10 per cent below their ideal weight range. The tables produced by the Metropolitan Life Insurance Company have been widely used. Note that the original purpose of these tables was for commercial use in assessing actuarial risk in people taking out life insurance policies. They were produced by recording the height and weight of a large number of life insurance applicants and then relating initial weight to risk of dying (and thus a claim on the policy) in the succeeding years. These ideal ranges were those associated with the lowest death rates. People above or below these ranges (i.e underweight or overweight) had higher death rates.

The need for frame size measurements makes these tables relatively cumbersome and inconvenient to use. Many people find it difficult to decide which frame size category they should put themselves in. Listed below are the ideal weight ranges for a man of average height (5 ft 9 in or 1.75 m) depending upon his frame size:

> small frame – 142–151 lb (64.3–68.3 kg)
> medium frame – 148–160 lb (67–72.7 kg)
> large frame – 155–176 lb (70.1–79.6 kg)

This means that a man of this height who weighed 170 lb could regard himself as either well within the ideal range or 20 lb over it depending upon his decision about his frame size. There are objective measures of frame size such as wrist circumference and elbow breadth which are not difficult to measure in a clinic or laboratory but they are not convenient measures for self-assessment.

The Body Mass Index (BMI)

In recent years the **Body Mass Index (BMI)** has become the usual routine way of assessing fatness. The BMI is the weight (in kilograms) divided by the height (in metres) squared.

$$BMI = \frac{weight\ (kg)}{height\ (m)^2}$$

For example, take a person who weighs 65 kg and is 1.78 m tall:

$$BMI = \frac{65}{1.78 \times 1.78} = 20.5$$

For those still used to the old imperial units then the same answer can be obtained using the following formula:

$$BMI = \frac{weight\ (pounds)}{height\ (inches)^2} \times 705$$

For example, take a person who is 5 ft 10 in (70 in) and weighs 143 lb (10 stone 3 lb):

$$BMI = \frac{143}{70 \times 70} \times 705 = 20.6$$

Table 1.2 a   Weights that represent key Body Mass Index values at different heights in metric units

Height(m)	Weight for BMI(kg)				
	17.5	**20**	**25**	**30**	**40**
1.45	36.8	42.1	52.6	63.1	84.1
1.47	37.8	43.2	54.0	64.8	86.0
1.50	39.4	45.0	56.3	67.5	90.0
1.52	40.4	46.2	57.8	69.3	92.4
1.55	42.0	48.1	60.1	72.1	96.1
1.57	43.1	49.3	61.6	73.9	98.6
1.60	44.8	51.2	64.0	76.8	102.4
1.63	46.5	53.1	66.4	79.7	106.3
1.65	47.6	54.5	68.1	81.7	108.9
1.68	49.4	56.4	70.6	84.7	112.9
1.70	50.6	57.8	72.3	86.7	115.6
1.73	52.4	59.9	74.8	89.8	119.7
1.75	53.6	61.3	76.6	91.9	122.5
1.78	55.4	63.4	79.2	95.1	126.7
1.80	56.7	64.8	81.0	97.2	129.6
1.83	58.6	67.0	83.8	100.5	134.0
1.85	59.9	68.5	85.6	102.7	136.9
1.88	61.9	70.7	88.4	106.0	141.4

1.90	63.2	72.2	90.3	108.3	144.4
1.93	65.2	74.5	93.1	111.7	149.0
1.95	66.5	76.1	95.1	114.1	152.1
1.98	68.6	78.4	98.0	117.6	156.8
2.00	70.0	80.0	100.0	120.0	160.0

Table 1.2 b The weights that represent key Body Mass Index values at different heights in imperial units

Height ft/in	Weight for BMI (pounds)				
	17.5	**20**	**25**	**30**	**40**
4'9"	81	93	116	139	185
4'10"	83	95	119	143	191
4'11"	87	99	124	148	198
5'	89	102	127	153	204
5'1"	93	106	132	159	212
5'2"	95	109	136	163	217
5'3"	99	113	141	169	226
5'4"	103	117	146	176	234
5'5"	105	120	150	180	240
5'6"	109	124	156	187	249
5'7"	112	127	159	191	255
5'8"	115	132	165	198	264
5'9"	118	135	169	203	270
5'10"	122	140	175	210	279
5'11"	125	143	179	214	286
6'	129	148	185	222	296
6'1"	132	151	189	226	302
6'2"	136	156	195	234	312
6'3"	139	159	199	239	318
6'4"	144	164	205	246	329
6'5"	147	168	210	252	335
6'6"	151	173	216	259	346
6'7"	154	176	221	265	353

NB   1 stone = 14 pounds

When tested on groups of ordinary adults, BMI is found to be a surprisingly good predictor of body fat content. In some studies, it is almost as good as several of the sophisticated 'hi-tech' laboratory methods of measuring fatness. Nevertheless, it relies upon the assumption that at any given height, differences in body weight are largely due to differences in fatness and so for groups like body builders who may be heavy but lean, and elderly people who may be relatively light but fat, it gives a flawed estimate of fatness. Even with 'normal' young and middle-aged adults, it is not a precise measure of an individual's degree of fatness. It is a simple, convenient and practically useful *guide* to the fatness of most adults. Tables 1.2 a and b show the weights that represent key Body Mass Index values at different heights in metric and imperial units respectively.

People can be put into categories according to their BMI – Table 1.3 shows the BMI categorisation system now used internationally. These standard ranges are useful rough indicators for self-assessment and for doctors. They also make it easy to estimate and compare the prevalence of the overweight and the obese in populations.

Table 1.3   The internationally recognised classification of people by Body Mass Index (BMI)

BMI range	Classification
under 20	underweight
20 – 25	ideal range
25 – 30	overweight
over 30	obese
over 40	severely obese

The following classification system has been widely used in the USA. It is included for completeness and because it is still widely referred to in America.

BMI – Men	Classification	BMI – Women
under 20.7	underweight	under 19.1
20.7 – 26.4	normal	19.1 – 25.8
26.4 – 27.8	marginally overweight	25.8 – 27.3
27.8 – 31.1	overweight	27.3 – 32.2
31.1 – 45.4	severely overweight	32.2 – 44.8
over 45.4	morbid obesity	over 44.8

A major advantage of the system shown in Table 1.2 is its simplicity – a small number of ranges, whole round numbers and the same ranges for use with both sexes. Making such choices to aid simplicity inevitably means that one has sacrificed some accuracy and sensitivity. The ranges should be regarded as a general guide rather than absolute cut-off points. Small differences in BMI are still small even if one happens to be above and one below a borderline.

The cut-off points given in Table 1.3 are now widely used in the USA and in Europe. However, until recently, different cut-off points have been taken to indicate obesity in the USA (also shown in Table 1.3) i.e. a BMI of over 27.8 for men and over 27.3 for women and so several tables and figures in this book that present American data use these alternative cut-off points for the definition of overweight/obesity. Apart from these instances, **overweight**, in this book, refers to a BMI of over 25 and **obese** to a BMI of over 30.

Other ways of measuring body fatness

There are several other ways of estimating body fatness that are more sophisticated and theoretically more accurate than BMI. However, in unskilled or careless hands they may be much less accurate than the simpler BMI and may do little more than generate random numbers. These methods may be used to give the illusion of precise and sophisticated assessment and so inflate the fee that can be charged by the assessor.

Skinfold calipers

Skinfold thickness measured with skinfold calipers can be used to estimate fatness. The thickness of the skinfold will be largely dependent upon the amount of fat stored beneath the skin. People store much of their fat directly beneath their skin and it is assumed that the amount of this subcutaneous fat stored at certain specified sites will give an indication of the total amount of fat in the body.

The thickness of the skinfold at various defined body sites is measured and the sum of these skinfolds is determined. A calibration table or chart will give estimates of the body fatness from the sum of these skinfold thicknesses.

Although this is a more direct way of estimating fatness than BMI it does have a number of important disadvantages, such as those listed below.

- It is a relatively time-consuming method and subjects must undress to have their skinfolds measured.
- It requires considerable skill and care to obtain accurate and reliable skinfold measures.
- The conversion of skinfold thickness into an estimate of body fat content is an approximation, not least because there is considerable genetic and racial variation in the distribution of body fat.

If you are being assessed in this way then you should expect your assessor to take care to locate the chosen subcutaneous sites accurately, use at least three sites for measurement, use good quality, metal calipers and to take repeat measurements.

Body density

This method relies upon the fact that the density of fat is less than that of lean tissue. If one assumes that lean tissue has an average density of 1.1 kg/l and fat has a density of 0.9 kg/l, then measurement of whole body density enables one to estimate the proportion of fat and lean in the body. The principle is simple but the technical procedures required to obtain accurate values are quite elaborate. To calculate the body's density one has to measure its weight and its volume:

$$\text{density} = \frac{\text{weight}}{\text{volume}}$$

Volume is measured by comparing the weight of the body in air and its weight when fully immersed in water – the difference between these two values is the weight of water displaced by the body and this allows one to calculate its volume and hence the volume of the body (using Archimedes principle). This method is unsuitable for routine use but it has traditionally been used as the reference method to calibrate other methods.

Bioelectrical impedance

This method of measuring body composition is now being used in many health centres and fitness clubs and as the cost of the device falls and its operation becomes ever simpler, so its use will grow. It relies upon the fact that fatty tissue is a much poorer conductor of electricity than lean tissue. Electrodes are placed on one of the subject's hands and feet, a current is generated by the machine's battery in one limb, passes through the body and is picked up by the electrode on the other limb. The machine uses the resistance to the current or the 'impedance' to estimate lean body mass and body fat. If the subject's age, sex, height and weight are keyed in, this machine gives a rapid prediction of the amount and percentage of fat in the body.

How prevalent are overweight and obesity?

Britain and America

The majority of adults in Britain and America have BMIs above the optimal range (20–25) and the number of overweight and obese people is rising rapidly (see Figures 1.1a and 1.1b). These figures do not allow easy comparison of the prevalence of overweight/obesity in Britain and the USA because of the different cut-off points used, but prevalence is higher in America and around 60 per cent of American adults have BMIs that are over 25.

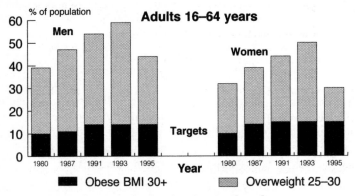

1.1a Prevalence of obesity in England

Data source: The Health Survey for England 1991, 1993 and 1995. London: HMSO

The governments of both countries have set targets for reducing the prevalence of obesity:

■ In England, *The Health of the Nation* target for obesity is that by the year 2005 no more than 6 per cent of men and 8 per cent of women should be clinically obese (BMI over 30). This was the estimated prevalence of obesity in 1980.

■ In the equivalent American document, *Healthy People 2000*, the stated objective is that by the year 2000, no more than 20 per cent of Americans should have BMIs that exceed 27.8 for men and 27.3 for women.

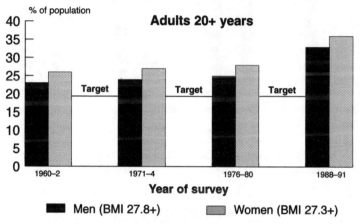

1.1b   Prevalence of obesity in the USA
Data source: Kuczmarski R J *et al* 1994. *Journal of the American Medical Association* 272, 205–211.

These targets are likely to be missed by very large margins. The long-term upward trend in prevalence of obesity has accelerated in both countries in the last 10–15 years. In England, in 1995, over 15 per cent of men and 16.5 per cent of women were obese and on current trends, levels are likely to be three times the target values in 2005. Figure 1.1b indicates that in 1988–91, 33 per cent of American adults had BMIs in excess of the threshold values and by the year 2000, the number of people exceeding these thresholds is likely to be around twice the 20 per cent target value.

Other countries

Figure 1.2 shows a comparison of the rates of obesity in four northern European countries. The Netherlands and especially Sweden seem to have lower rates of obesity than Britain and Germany (and thus also the USA). Rates seem to be increasing in all four countries but the rate of increase in Sweden is slow.

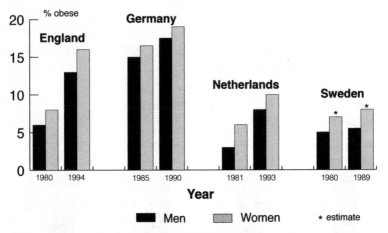

1.2   Rates of obesity (BMI 30+) in Europe
Data source: Obesity Research Information Service

Sweden is an affluent industrialised country and yet the prevalence of obesity seems to be less than half that seen in Britain and America and is only rising slowly. Prevalence of obesity in England in 1980 was less than half what it is today. These figures are paradoxically both alarming and encouraging for Britons and Americans. Alarming, because unless the trend is halted or reversed, in a few decades time, it may become rare to see a middle-aged American or Briton who is not overweight. A very substantial proportion of these populations will be carrying enough excess weight to seriously impair their health and quality of life. Encouraging, because it is clear that relatively low levels of obesity are not incompatible with an affluent and industrialised lifestyle. If English and American people adopted the dietary and lifestyle practices of England prior to 1980, or followed current Swedish practices, then levels of obesity should fall towards the government targets.

Looking beyond Europe and America, obesity is becoming an increasing problem amongst some relatively affluent urban populations in developing countries. In some of these countries, one has the contrast between widespread and increasing obesity in affluent sections of the urban population and malnutrition and starvation in poorer sections of the population.

Which Britons and Americans get fat?

Effect of age on obesity prevalence

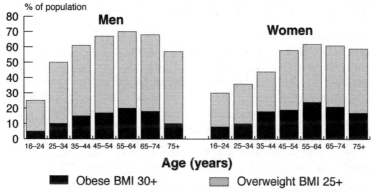

1.3a Effect of age on obesity prevalence in England
Data source: The Health Survey for England 1993. London: HMSO

Figures 1.3a and 1.3b show the prevalence of overweight and obesity in different age groups in England and the USA. The trends in both countries are very similar; for both sexes, the prevalence seems to peak in late middle age and then start to fall. Increasing levels of chronic illness and disability in the elderly partly explains the declining levels of obesity in older age groups. There may also be a general tendency for people to lose weight towards the end of their life.

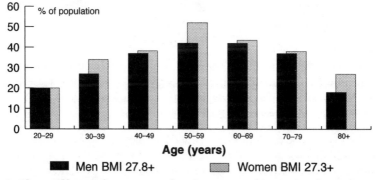

1.3b Effect of age on obesity prevalence in the USA
Data source: Kuczmarski R J et al, 1994. *Journal of the American Medical Association* 272, 205–211

Obesity is most prevalent amongst middle-aged people, more than two thirds of middle-aged Britons and Americans are overweight or obese.

Ethnicity and obesity prevalence

There are large differences in obesity rates among different ethnic groups living in the same country. This suggests varying genetic susceptibility to obesity between ethnic groups. Cultural/lifestyle differences also contribute to this varying susceptibility to obesity. Socioeconomic inequalities may also be a factor, for example, the poverty rate among black Americans is three times that among whites and obesity rate is strongly affected by social class (see below).

In Britain, central obesity (i.e. with a concentration of fat in the abdomen) is more common amongst people of South Asian origin than it is in the white population. These groups are assumed to be genetically susceptible to storing large amounts of fat in the abdominal region and this may be a factor in their high risk of diabetes and heart disease (see Chapter 2).

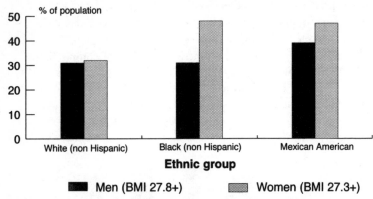

1.4   Prevalence of obesity by ethnic group in the USA
Data source: Kuczmarski R J et al, 1994. *Journal of the American Medical Association* 272, 205–211

In the USA, some tribes of native Americans have rates of obesity in their adult populations that are more than double that in the white population. Figure 1.4 shows how the obesity prevalence varies between ethnic groups in the USA. Around 39 per cent of Mexican American men and around 48 per cent of both Mexican American and black American women had BMIs in excess of the threshold values compared to only about 32 per cent of white American men and women.

There are racial differences in obesity prevalence. In Britain, abdominal obesity is particularly prevalent amongst people of South Asian origin (i.e. from India, Pakistan, Sri Lanka and Bangladesh). In the USA, obesity is particularly prevalent amongst native Americans, Mexican Americans and black American women.

Social class

Obesity is a major public health problem in most wealthy industrialised countries whereas in poorer countries obesity will be largely confined to the most affluent sections of society. Poor people in poor countries struggle to obtain enough to eat and are likely to have to do hard physical work to survive – obesity is improbable under these circumstances. In the industrialised countries, obesity is no longer a symbol of wealth and success but is actually more prevalent amongst the lower social classes – the stereotype of obesity being largely the province of the wealthy businessman who overindulges in costly expense account lunches is inaccurate. In a large English survey, the lowest average BMIs and the lowest rates of obesity were found in men and women of the highest social class and the highest average BMI and highest rates of obesity found in those in the lowest social class (see Figure 1.5).

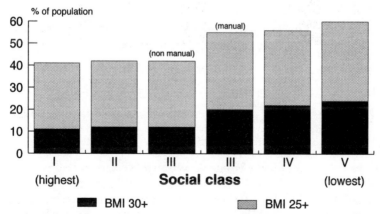

1.5   Prevalence of obesity by social class in English women
Data source: The Health Survey for England 1993. London: HMSO 1995.

In industrialised countries, obesity is more prevalent amongst the lower socioeconomic groups whereas in the poorest countries of the world only the relatively affluent have the opportunity to get fat.

How much food do I need?

Calories, kilocalories and kilojoules

Throughout this book, calories are used as the units of energy. A **calorie** is actually a very small unit and so in nutrition the term calorie is used to mean a thousand calories (i.e. strictly a kilocalorie, kcal). If readers see energy expressed in **kilojoules** (kJ) then:1 calorie = 4.2 kJ (To roughly convert calories to kilojoules multiply by 4.) Thus a thousand calories (i.e. strictly 1000 kilocalories) is 4200 kilojoules.

Average energy requirements

Table 1.4 shows the current estimated average daily energy requirements for older (above the age of 11) children and adults in the UK and America. Daily energy requirements rise during childhood and peak in adolescence. Children's smaller size is the sole reason that their energy requirements are lower than those of adults. In fact, children have higher energy requirements per unit of body weight because they are more active, are growing and have faster metabolic rates. For example, a two-year-old child may only weigh about a fifth of an adult's weight but requires around half the amount of energy required by an adult.

Table 1.4 The estimated average daily calorie requirements for older children and adults in the UK and USA

Age group (years)		UK	USA
11–14	boys	2220	2500
	girls	1845	2200
15–18	boys	2755	3000
	girls	2110	2200
19–50	men	2550	2900
	women	1940	2200
51–59	men	2550	2300
	women	1900	1900
60–64	men	2380	2300
	women	1900	1900
75+	men	2100	2300
	women	1810	1900

Energy requirements decline in late middle-age and old age for two main reasons:

- people tend to become less active as they get older;
- resting metabolic rate falls because elderly people have less muscle (probably as a consequence of inactivity).

If elderly people eat less food because of their reduced energy needs, then they will probably also take in less of the essential nutrients. Their need for these nutrients does not generally decline and in some instances may actually increase. Elderly people, particularly very inactive elderly people, are thus more prone to nutrient deficiencies unless their diet is rich in nutrients. Similar arguments would apply to people on low calorie diets.

Two important points about the values in Table 1.4 should be borne in mind. Firstly, they are *average* values and so one would expect about half of all individuals to require more and half less than these values. Any individual's exact energy requirements will depend upon their size and body composition, their activity level, their state of health, their genetic make-up etc. This is an important point to remember when using these values to predict the energy needs or to judge the energy intakes of individuals. The second point is that they are *estimated* requirements, i.e. they are the 'best guess' of a committee of nutrition experts. This point is well illustrated by the differences between the American and British values in the table.

How are these average calorie needs estimated?

Basal metabolic rate (BMR) is the energy expended by a rested and fasted person lying down in a warm room. It is the minimum expenditure in a conscious person and represents the energy required to keep the essential systems of the body functioning. If BMR is measured in many hundreds of individuals then it is found that within age and sex groups, BMR tends to rise in a predictable way with increasing body weight. This makes it possible to derive equations that predict the *average* BMR of a group of people of known age and sex from their average weight. The expert committees who derived the values in Table 1.4 made assumptions about the average body weight of subjects within each age and sex band and then used equations to predict the average BMR.

Then, to convert the BMR into an estimate of the total energy requirement, one needs to multiply the BMR by some factor to allow for the level of physical activity, this is called the **Physical Activity Level, (PAL)**. The values in Table 1.4 represent between 1.4 × BMR (e.g. in British adults aged 19–50 years) to 1.7 × BMR (e.g. in American boys aged 11–14 years). Most of the differences between the American and British values in Table 1.4 represent differences in the PAL multiples used by the American and British experts; Americans also tend to be a little heavier than Britons.

For example, the British expert panel assumed an average weight of 74 kg for men aged 19–50 years and then used the following equation to predict the average BMR:

BMR (calories per day) = 15.1 × weight(kg) + 692

So for an average weight of 74 kg:

average BMR = (15.1 × 74) + 692

average BMR = 1809 calories per day

They multiplied this by 1.4 to allow for the Physical Activity Level of a man who is sedentary in both his work (e.g. office worker) and leisure (e.g. spends most of his time watching TV). After rounding, this gives an estimated energy requirement of 2550 calories per day.

The US panel used a similar equation to predict the BMR of a typical man aged 25–50 years but they assumed an average weight of 79 kg and used a PAL multiple of 1.6. This is why the USA figures in Table 1.4 are higher than the UK figures.

Can I estimate my own energy needs?

It is possible to estimate one's own calorie needs but this process is crude and is particularly sensitive to errors in classifying one's activity level.

For adults under 50, one assumes that at rest, each kilogram of body uses 0.9 calories per hour in women (1.0 in men). So, the BMR of a 60 kg woman would be estimated at:

60 × 0.9 × 24 = 1296 calories per day

To estimate this woman's daily energy expenditure, one must now multiply this by an appropriate PAL factor. Table 1.5 gives some PAL multiples that may be appropriate for different activity levels. Let us assume that our woman is a teacher who walks a fair bit at work but does not regularly participate in active pursuits in her free time. Her total energy should lie within the range:

BMR $\times$ 1.4–1.6 (i.e. 1814 to 2074 calories per day)

Table 1:5   Multiples of BMR (Physical Activity Level, PAL) that can be used to estimate total energy expenditure at varying activity levels

Activity level	PAL multiple Men	Women	Description
Sedentary	1.25–1.4	1.25–1.35	Mostly sitting and riding e.g. sedentary office worker who drives to work. Elderly housebound person.
Light activity	1.5–1.7	1.4–1.6	E.g. a teacher who walks around a fair amount whilst working.
Moderate activity	1.65–1.8	1.5–1.7	E.g. office worker who takes regular exercise, say, jogs five times a week.
Heavy activity	1.9–2.2	1.8–2.0	Someone whose work involves sustained heavy manual work e.g. digging with a pickaxe and shovel.
Exceptional	2.3–2.45	2.1–2.3	Professional or other serious athletes in the training season.

How much food do these energy requirements represent?

Our dietary energy comes from carbohydrates, fats and protein (plus alcohol for some people). One gram of fat yields roughly the same number of calories whatever type of fat it is and the same is true for carbohydrates and proteins. Thus:

■ one gram of fat yields 9 calories (whether it is saturated or unsaturated fat);

■ one gram of carbohydrate yields about 4 calories (whether it is sugar or starch);

■ one gram of protein yields 4 calories;

■ one gram of alcohol yields 7 calories.

Table 1.6 shows how much fat, carbohydrate and protein the British and American estimates of the average energy requirements of young adults represents. The figures in Table 1.6 look very small when one considers the weight of food that most of us actually consume in a day – somewhere around a pound (0.5 kg) of these nutrients is enough for most adults. Of course, when we eat food then these nutrients are diluted to varying extents by other things, especially water and dietary fibre. Just to illustrate the large effect that water content can have on the energy yield of foods, grapes yield only 60 calories per 100 g but if they are dried to make raisins then this increases to 246 calories per 100 g.

Table 1:6   The amount of carbohydrate, fat and protein that the USA and UK estimates the calorie requirements of adults represents

Group	Estimate (kcal)	Weight of nutrients*		
		Carbohydrate	+ Fat +	Protein
UK males	2550	340 g + (c. 12 oz	100 g + c. 3.5 oz	94 g c. 3.5 oz)
UK females	1940	260 g + (c. 9.5 oz	75 g + c. 2.5 oz	73 g c. 2.5 oz)
US males	2900	390 g + (c. 14 oz	115 g + c. 4 oz	100 g c. 3.5 oz)
US females	2200	300 g + (c. 10.5 oz	85 g + c. 3 oz	78 g c. 3 oz)

*Assumed 35 per cent of calories come from fat, 50 per cent from carbohydrate and the rest from protein

The energy yield per unit weight of foods (e.g. calories per 100 g) is referred to as its **energy density**. High water content clearly reduces the energy density of foods. High fat content greatly increases energy density because a given weight of fat yields more than twice as many calories as the same amount of either protein or carbohydrate. A gram of pure sugar yields only about 40 per cent of the calories of a gram of a pure fat such as vegetable oil. Table 1.7 illustrates the dramatic effect that changes in fat content can have on the energy density of foods or meals. Adding small amounts of fat to bulky food can have a disproportionate effect upon the total energy yield. For example, adding a layer of butter or margarine to a slice of bread may increase the energy content by 80 per cent and adding a tablespoon of mayonnaise to a mixed salad results in a six fold rise in the energy yield.

Table 1:7   The effect of adding typical portions of fats to typical portions of some foods

Food	calories	% increase
slice of bread	75	
+ butter/margarine	134	79
jacket potato	147	
+ butter/margarine	221	50
boiled potatoes	120	
chips/french fries	379	216
pork chop – lean	180	
lean and fat	348	93
lean steak	260	
lean and fat	338	68
skimmed milk	64	
whole milk	129	102
chicken meat	121	
meat and skin	184	52
fruit pie	223	
+ double cream	380	70
mixed salad	28	
+ oil/vinegar	87	211
mixed salad	28	
+ mayonnaise	166	493

Below, I have selected three fairly ordinary meals or snacks and calculated their energy value. Thus, someone who ate the high calorie breakfast and lunch and the high calorie burger meal during the course of a day would be taking in almost exactly 3000 calories even without allowing for any additional drinks or snacks – sedentary men and most women would gain weight on this sort of diet. This does not appear to be a vast amount of food. Most people, certainly most men, could probably manage to eat this in the course of any given day – one does not have to gorge oneself on vast quantities of food to gain weight.

For each of these three meals I have also given an alternative lower calorie version. These are not intended to be recommendations but to show that relatively modest changes to meals can greatly affect their energy yield, and that it is possible to reduce energy intake without totally changing the pattern of eating. Someone eating the low calorie versions of the breakfast, lunch and burger meal would be consuming under 1750 calories (or 1650 calories if they chose the very low calorie breakfast) – most men and many large and/or moderately active women might expect to lose at least some weight on such a diet. This is still quite a substantial amount of food, indeed in terms of crude bulk it is not much different from the high calorie day's food – it is possible for a reasonably active person to eat three proper meals per day and stay slim or even lose weight gradually if they make the right sort of choices. One dieter in a family can adapt a normal family diet into a reducing diet.

Note that the high calorie meal selections contain two-and-a-quarter times as much fat as the reduced calorie versions. In the high calorie meals around 39 per cent of all the calories come from fat whereas in the reduced calorie choices only 29 per cent come from fat (less than 27 per cent if the very low calorie breakfast is chosen). This gives an early indication that reducing fat intake is a key factor in reducing total calorie intake.

High calorie version	**Reduced calorie version**
Breakfast	
734 calories	536 calories*
Cornflakes (with whole milk and 1 tsp sugar)	Cornflakes (with semi-skimmed milk and 1 tsp sugar)
glass orange juice	glass orange juice
coffee (with whole milk and 1tsp sugar)	coffee (with semi-skimmed milk)

| Two toasted 'pop tarts' | 2 slices toast with 10g butter/margarine and 20g jam |

* This reduced calorie breakfast could be reduced still further if skimmed milk and low fat spread were substituted and if the cornflakes were eaten without added sugar - such a breakfast would yield only 458 calories.

Packed lunch

959 calories	561 calories
4 slices bread with	4 slices bread with
10 g butter/margarine	5 g butter/margarine
60 g cheddar cheese	60 g low fat cottage cheese
1 tbsp coleslaw	tomato and cucumber
Mars bar	apple and banana

Burger bar meal

1310 calories	631 calories
large fries (4.3 oz)	small fries (2.4 oz)
quarterpounder with cheese	quarterpounder
milk shake	diet cola

Conclusions

■ The Body Mass Index (BMI) is the most common way of assessing weight status. It is the weight in kilograms divided by the height in metres squared.

■ Adults whose BMI is in the 25–30 range are classified as overweight and those whose BMI is above 30 classified as obese.

■ In industrialised countries, obesity is most prevalent amongst the middle-aged and those in the lower socioeconomic groups.

■ There is a considerable ethnic variation in obesity rates and body fat distribution.

■ Expert committees in industrialised countries publish estimates of the energy needs of the average person according to age and sex group but any individual's energy needs depend upon many factors such as their size, body composition and particularly their level of physical activity.

■ It is possible for most people to eat recognisably normal meals and still lose weight by making sensible modifications and especially by reducing the fatty components of the meal. Weight loss is not incompatible with a normal family diet!

2 CONSEQUENCES OF BEING OVERWEIGHT OR OBESE

Scope of the chapter

In this chapter I will discuss the health and other consequences of being underweight, overweight or obese and try to explain why being too fat increases the risks of illness and premature death. I will discuss how factors such as age, sex and the distribution of body fat affect the health risks of excess fatness and try to give some criteria to help readers decide whether they should take active steps to try to lose weight.

Is it fine to be fat?

In 1976, even before the recent surge in obesity rates, a committee of British health experts unanimously concluded that:

> 'obesity is a hazard to health and a detriment to well-being ... it is common enough to constitute one of the most important medical and public health problems of our time.'
>
> *Research on Obesity*. Report of the DHSS/MRC Group.
> Complied by WPT James (1976) London: HMSO

Since the beginning of the twentieth century, records kept by life insurance companies have suggested that being substantially overweight increases the risk of premature death – increased insurance premiums are one undeniable disadvantage of being obese. Figure 2.1 shows that Americans who are overweight when they take out life insurance are more likely to die during the following years than those of 'average' weight. The risk accelerates upwards as the amount of excess weight increases and seems to be greater in men than in women. These general findings have been repeated many times, including some studies that have used random population samples rather than unrepresentative life insurance

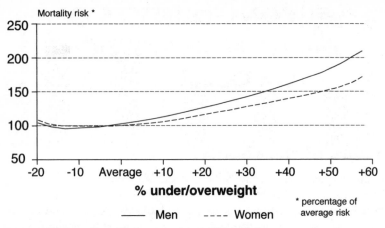

2.1 Effect of weight on mortality risk

samples. Factors such as the age range of the subjects, their sex and whether or not they include smokers affects the precise shape of the graph and thus the apparent 'ideal' BMI it suggests.

Effect of age on the risk posed by excess weight

The risks of being obese seem to be higher in younger people. In very obese men, mortality was found to be 12 times greater than normal in those who were aged 25–34 years, but only three times greater than normal in those aged 45–54 years. (Of course, the risk is 12 times a very small number in the young men but three times a bigger number in the older men.)

Figure 2.2 is constructed from life insurance records and indicates that the 'ideal' BMI (the one with the lowest risk of death) tends to drift upwards with age. In women in their twenties, then, the BMI at which the death rate was lowest was only 19.5 whereas in those in their sixties it had risen to 27.3 (i.e. overweight).

Several studies in different countries have reported that in older people, say over 65, being moderately overweight seems to be associated with increased life expectancy in marked contrast to the reduced life expectancy consistently found in overweight or obese young people. As an extreme example, one study in Finland found a steady increase in five year survival

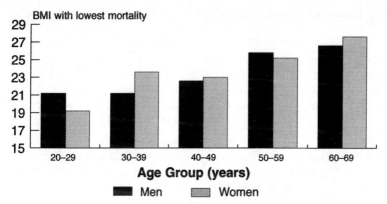

2.2   Effect of age on the risks of being overweight
Data source: Andres R et al, 1985. *Journal of Internal Medicine* 103,
1031–1033.

rate with increasing BMI in people aged over 85. The highest survival was
recorded in those with BMIs of over 28.

A partial explanation for this apparent reversal of risk with age is that, in
elderly people, low body weight may be a strong indicator of existing poor
health. There may also be a general tendency for people to lose weight as
they approach the end of their life. Average BMI and rates of obesity
certainly decline in those aged over 60 (see Chapter 1). Health and social
problems that can reduce food intake and lead to nutritional deficiencies
are more common in the elderly. Extra stores of fat and nutrients may act
as a buffer during these adverse circumstances.

This does not mean that all attempts at weight control should be
abandoned in later life. Some changes in behaviour that may lead to
weight reduction, such as taking more exercise or eating less fat, can be
justified on wider health grounds. Obesity will reduce mobility and will
worsen problems like diabetes, hypertension or arthritis. Nevertheless,
perhaps the 'ideal' upper weight limit could be relaxed for elderly people
particularly if they are healthy, mobile and do not have a condition that is
aggravated by being overweight. On purely health grounds, is dieting
desirable for healthy and mobile elderly people (those over 70) whose
BMI is below 30? 'Improving' the diet and encouraging activity should be
the health priority rather than changes in body weight *per se*. Of course,
elderly people may still wish to try to lose weight for reasons of self-
esteem – the reason why most younger people diet.

Is being underweight a health hazard?

Figure 2.1 suggests some increase in death rate both in those who are overweight and underweight, i.e. there is a so-called J-shaped curve. This J-curve has been found in many other studies. In one study, BMI was measured in 1.8 million Norwegians and related to deaths over a ten-year period – life expectancy was reduced in those with very low and very high BMI with the highest life expectancy found in the BMI 21–26 range.

The higher death rate at low BMI has usually been explained by suggesting that being underweight is often an indicator of poor health, an early indication of some undiagnosed condition, or the result of alcohol, tobacco or drug abuse. Smoking, in particular, is known to depress body weight and is also a cause of much ill-health and many premature deaths. Figure 2.3, from a study of 115,000 American female nurses, shows a typical J-curve of mortality against BMI. However, Figure 2.3 also shows the results from this study when the following 'corrections' were made:

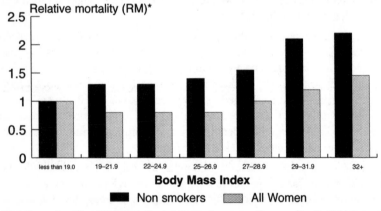

■ Non smokers   ▨ All Women

*Rm is the number of times higher the death rate is than for the corresponding group when the BMI is less than 19, e.g. if the RM for a group of non smokers is two this means that there are twice as many deaths as in non smokers with BMIs of less than 19.

2.3 BMI and mortality in women: the effects of smoking
Data source: Manson J E *et al*, 1995. *The New England Journal of Medicine* 333, 677–685.

■ those who died within the first four years were excluded (i.e. those already in poor health when the study started);

■ only those whose weight was stable at the start of the study were included (recent unintentional weight loss is an indicator of ill-health);

■ only women who had never smoked were included (smoking damages health and lowers body weight).

The J-curve disappears when these people are excluded. The increase in death rate with increasing BMI is also more pronounced.

Figure 2.3 offers reassurance for otherwise healthy women who are slightly underweight provided that they eat well and have not experienced any recent unexplained weight loss. There is, however, no doubt that being seriously underweight due to self-starvation is a serious health hazard as seen in the consequences of anorexia nervosa which I list later in the chapter. Most obviously, a minimum amount of body fat is essential for fertility and successful reproduction – women who are very underweight stop menstruating and become infertile. Puberty is delayed in underweight girls, and underweight women are more likely to have an underweight baby, especially if they have had fertility treatment.

Figure 2.3 should not be used to suggest even lower BMI targets. The relationship between BMI and mortality seems to be fairly flat for BMIs between 19 and 27. On purely health grounds, if people don't smoke, don't drink excessively, take regular exercise and eat a reasonably healthy diet then one can be fairly relaxed about BMIs certainly up to 27. Of course, such people are also less likely to be overweight in the first place.

Are eating disorders a consequence of our obsession with dieting?

Around two million people in the USA may suffer from either **anorexia nervosa** or **bulimia nervosa**. The term **eating disorders** also includes many other people who have some symptoms of these conditions but fall short of the formal diagnostic criteria.

Anorexia nervosa affects mainly females who typically are: white; age 15–25 years; from middle and upper class families; well-educated; and, with a good knowledge of nutrition. Cases do occur in men (about a twentieth of the frequency in women), and in other age, social and racial groups. As it becomes more common, so anorexia is radiating out from its traditional risk group. The characteristics of this disease are:

■ very low body weight;
■ intense fear of becoming fat even though underweight;
■ distorted body image – seeing themselves as fat even though emaciated;

- lack of menstrual periods;
- frequently, use of laxatives or induced vomiting;
- often intense physical activity, unlike other victims of starvation.

Victims of the disease may also try to conceal their eating habits and physical emaciation from relatives and friends. They may wear loose clothing; avoid social eating situations; eat very slowly; only eat low calorie foods; only pretend to eat; induce vomiting after eating; and take laxatives in the mistaken belief that this will get rid of calories.

Significant numbers of sufferers die as a result of anorexia or its complications – they literally starve themselves to death. The consequences of anorexia are largely due to starvation and are listed below:

- wasting of lean tissue and vital organs;
- reduced growth in young people;
- depressed immune function and increased susceptibility to infections;
- lack of menstruation, infertility and loss of sex drive;
- reduced bone density (osteoporosis) and increased risk of fractures, especially stress fractures in anorexic athletes;
- slow healing of wounds;
- reduced physical work capacity and impaired performance in dancers and athletes;
- shrinkage of heart muscle, irregular heart rhythm and risk of heart failure;
- reduced digestive and absorption capability in the gut often leading to diarrhoea;
- hypothermia;
- abnormal (excess) amounts of body hair in women;
- insomnia, changes in personality and brain function.

Bulimia nervosa is characterised by recurrent bouts of binge eating. A binge is usually followed by compensatory behaviour, for example, induced vomiting, intense exercise, fasting or purging. Bulimia occurs in people whose weight is within the normal range and as they are guilty and secretive about their behaviour, this makes it difficult to diagnose. Bulimic people share the anorexic's morbid fear of fatness and distortion of body image. Bulimia would be diagnosed if bouts of bingeing and compensatory behaviour occurred regularly and persistently in a person who was not very underweight but who was preoccupied with their shape and weight.

Does dieting cause eating disorders?

These eating disorders have become much more common in recent decades. They seem to be triggered by social pressures upon young people to be lean and to diet. Many bulimic patients have a history of cycles of weight loss and regain or 'yo-yo dieting'. Eating disorders are more common amongst women for whom thinness is a career requirement such as models, ballet dancers, airline stewardesses, gymnasts and other athletes. In male athletes and ballet dancers, eating disorders are almost as common as in women despite their general rarity in men.

In some classical studies, normal, healthy young male volunteers were partially starved for several months. This starvation greatly affected their personalities and behaviour. During starvation their scores on personality tests deteriorated and some became indicative of psychiatric illness. During the starvation period, they developed eating behaviours typically seen in anorexics. During rehabilitation several men were inclined to binge. Some of these changes in food-related behaviour, including bouts of dieting, persisted long after the experiment was over.

These observations suggest that eating disorders may be triggered by social and cultural conditions that require young women, in particular, to be thin. The dieting itself may, in susceptible individuals, cause some of the unusual and irrational behaviour seen in anorexics. Initially, praise for weight loss and leanness acts as a reward for anorexic behaviour, so encouraging repetition and learning. In someone whose self-esteem is low and who feels dominated by others, then this ability to control one aspect of their life may also encourage anorexic behaviour.

These diseases are essentially confined to affluent societies where food is plentiful; societies where there is a conflict between the ready availability of tempting energy rich foods, low requirement for physical activity and yet strong social pressures to be lean. As the affluent populations in the Western world have got fatter, so the image of the ideal body shape seems to have got thinner. One study showed that during the 1960s and 1970s the winners of American beauty contests and models in pin-up magazines got steadily thinner. The widening gap between the ideal that people aspire to and the practical reality is a recipe for despair.

How does obesity affect health and wellbeing?

I have listed below certain conditions which are caused or worsened by obesity and which contribute to the reduced life expectancy of obese people.

Heart and circulatory system
coronary heart disease;
strokes;
hypertension;
angina pectoris;
sudden death due to ventricular arrythmia (abnormal heart rhythm);
congestive heart failure;
varicose veins, haemorrhoids, swollen ankles, venous thrombosis.

Joints
osteoarthritis – knees.

Endocrine/metabolic
non-insulin dependent diabetes mellitus (maturity onset diabetes);
gout;
raised blood lipids including blood cholesterol;
gallstones.

Cancer
increased risk of cancer of the ovary, cervix (neck of the womb), breast and endometrium (lining of the womb).

Other
increased risk of pregnancy complications;
reduced fertility;
menstrual irregularities;
increased risk during anaesthesia and surgery;
reduced mobility, agility and increased risk of accidents;
adverse psychological, social and economic consequences (see later in the chapter).

Death rates from heart attacks, strokes, diabetes and certain cancers are particularly high in obese people.

Being overweight or obese increases several of the **risk factors** that are known to make people susceptible to heart disease and strokes. As people gain weight these risk factors tend to rise and they tend to fall during weight reduction i.e. weight gain, or the behaviours that lead to weight gain, directly cause these risk factor rises. Some examples are listed below.

■ Excessive weight gain raises blood pressure and increases risk of hypertension. Blood pressure tends to rise with BMI in all age and sex groups – in one large English survey, people with BMIs of over 30 had double the risk of having high blood pressure compared with those with BMIs of 20–25. Weight loss is one of the accepted ways of treating hypertension.

■ Obesity reduces our response to the hormone insulin and this can precipitate the milder, late-onset form of diabetes (**non insulin dependent diabetes mellitus**) which does not usually require insulin injections. Even this mild form of the disease has unpleasant symptoms and serious effects upon long-term health. Some immediate consequences are:
  – increased urine production;
  – increased thirst and drinking;
  – tiredness and lethargy;
  – blurred vision;
  – recurrent genitourinary tract infections

Some long-term consequences are:

  – increased risk of heart disease and strokes;
  – kidney failure (diabetic nephropathy);
  – damage to the retina of the eye (diabetic retinopathy);
  – cataracts;
  – loss of sensation due to nerve damage (diabetic neuropathy);
  – gangrene of feet and legs.

In experimental animals and human volunteers, deliberate overfeeding and weight gain reduces the response to insulin and this can precipitate diabetes. Insulin response increases during weight loss. Being moderately obese may increase the risk of subsequently developing diabetes by more than 10 fold. Weight loss is known to lessen the symptoms and consequences of this type of diabetes.

■ Obese people have increased blood cholesterol levels. High cholesterol is linked to increased risk of heart disease and strokes.

■ Obese people tend to have high blood uric acid levels. This causes the painful joint condition gout and increases the risk of heart disease. Weight loss reduces the symptoms of gout and lowers blood uric acid levels.

■ Obesity is associated with an increased tendency for blood to clot and form thromboses.

Much of the health risk of moderate levels of overweight can be accounted for by these increases in risk factor levels leading some to suggest that the direct health risks of mild obesity have been greatly exaggerated. It has been argued by some feminist writers that women, in particular, are thus persuaded to aim for unreasonably low target weights leading to low self-esteem and even to eating disorders in some susceptible women. Remember, however, that excessive fatness, or the behaviours that cause fatness, appear to cause the increase in these other risk factors. Risk factors increase as weight is gained and decrease during weight loss. Increases in risk factors seems to be one of the mechanisms by which obesity causes illness and death.

Obesity, disability and quality of life

Some of the problems listed on p.36 may cause considerable ill-health and disability, even though not often a direct cause of death. One Finnish study found that overweight people were much more likely to claim a disability pension than lean people. The authors concluded that being overweight was a major cause of disability in Finland. The effect of overweight on disability seemed to be more pronounced in women than in men and started at BMIs where the effect on death rate is small (25+ in women and 27+ in men).

One American study found that even moderately obese people were more likely than lean people to report problems in personal functioning, for example, in bathing, dressing, walking, climbing stairs and getting around their community. Those who were more severely affected had even more problems with personal functioning and they also admitted limitations in performing their occupational work, school work or housework.

Being obese not only means increased risk of premature death but also higher incidence of several non-fatal conditions, higher risk of disability and more chance of being unable to adequately perform the tasks of everyday living. Both the length of life and the expectations of life are lower in obese people.

Social, economic and psychological effects of obesity

Obesity is a social and economic handicap. Obese people are widely perceived as being weak, greedy, lazy and self-indulgent individuals who overeat because they lack willpower and to compensate for their emotional inadequacies. These attitudes to the obese are very pervasive and seem to become ingrained in early childhood. In one famous study, children as young as six years old rated pictures of obese children as less likeable than lean children and often less likeable than pictures of those with physical deformities. They attribute unpleasant characteristics to the obese children in the pictures – comments such as they are: lazy, dirty, stupid, ugly and that they are cheats and liars.

The obese are also the victims of practical discrimination. Acceptance rates for some US colleges were lower amongst obese applicants, even when their academic entry qualifications were the same. The obese are at a disadvantage in the labour market because many employers perceive obese people as undesirable employees.

A research group from the Harvard Medical School studied 10,000 young people living in Boston. They found that there were substantial social and economic disadvantages to being obese. After seven years, those women who were obese (average BMI 35) at the start of the study had completed fewer years at school, had lower household incomes, were more likely to be below the poverty line and were less likely to be married. Neither initial differences in socioeconomic status nor their performance in intelligence and aptitude tests could explain the differences between the social performance of lean and obese subjects. They seemed to be due to prejudice and discrimination. The prospects of those with chronic physical conditions such as asthma, diabetes or muscle and joint problems were not impaired – being obese was more of a socioeconomic handicap than a chronic physical disability. Another study has found that obese women were less likely than lean women to marry a man of a higher social class – obese women have impaired social as well as physical mobility! The social and economic disadvantages of being obese seem to be less in men than in women.

There is a widespread belief that psychological instability and psychiatric problems are more common in obese people. This probably contributes towards the prejudice and discrimination experienced by the obese. There is little objective evidence to support this. Most surveys report little or no difference in psychological functioning or in the prevalence of psychiatric disturbances between random samples of lean and obese people. 'Disparagement of body' image is the one psychological disturbance to which obese people are particularly prone. They see themselves as grotesque and ugly and feel that they are viewed with contempt by other people. This poor body image is seen particularly in girls and young women from the upper socioeconomic groupings and is probably related to the prejudice and discrimination that obese people experience.

Much of the discrimination against obese people seems to be unjustified by higher levels of physical incapacity or psychological disturbance and must therefore be classified as prejudice. Obese people may be unsuitable for jobs that are physically demanding but being overweight would not be a significant handicap in many sedentary occupations. The finding that obese young people fare worse than those with chronic physical disabilities seems to confirm that physical incapacity is not a major reason for their poor socioeconomic performance. In other areas of prejudice and discrimination, the civilised response has been to try to prevent or reduce it by education or even legislation, for example, discrimination against individuals on the basis of religion, sex or ethnicity are illegal in both the USA and much of Europe. Should we likewise consider active steps to counteract unjustified prejudice and discrimination against obese people? There have been several successful prosecutions of employers in the USA for unreasonably discriminating against obese employees or job applicants. A self-help organisation, the National Association to Aid Fat Americans (NAAFA), aims to help obese people view themselves positively and to lead fuller, happier lives.

Is all body fat the same?

Waist-to-hip ratio is a simple indicator of body fat distribution. It is the circumference of the body at the waist divided by the circumference around the hips. Excess fat deposited in the abdomen seems to be more detrimental to health than other fat. People who are obese and have a high waist-to-hip ratio (so-called 'apples') seem to be more at risk from the effects of their obesity than people who are equally obese but have a low waist-to-hip ratio ('pears').

Figure 2.4 shows that waist-to-hip ratio is higher in men than in women and tends to rise with age in both sexes, i.e. people tend to thicken around the waist as they get older – they develop 'middle-aged spread'. Ideally it is suggested that waist-to-hip ratio should be less than 0.8 for women and less than 0.95 (or even 0.9) for men. A BMI of 27 in a person with a high waist-to-hip ratio may carry more health risk than a BMI of 30 in someone with a low waist-to-hip ratio.

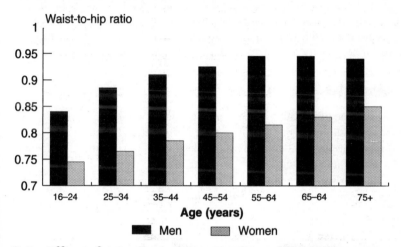

2.4 Effect of age on average waist-to-hip ratio
Data source: The Health Survey for England 1993. London: HMSO 1995

Large amounts of abdominal fat seem to predispose people to diabetes and heart disease. The increase in heart disease may be largely a consequence of the predisposition to diabetes. People of South Asian origin (from the Indian subcontinent) seem to be genetically prone to store more fat in their abdomens than Caucasians. At any given BMI, South Asians have a higher waist-to-hip ratio than Caucasians. This may partly explain the unexpectedly high prevalence of diabetes and heart disease seen in British Asians. In the UK, the prevalence of diabetes is around five times higher in South Asians than Caucasians and rates of heart disease about three times what one would expect.

Inactivity is thought to be strongly linked to a high waist-to-hip ratio as well as being linked to overweight and obesity generally. Heavy smokers and heavy drinkers have high waist-to-hip ratios and there is some evidence that these behaviours cause fat to be deposited in the abdomen.

To sum up

Waist-to-hip ratio rises with age in both sexes. High waist-to-hip ratio is a predictor of increased risk of death. It is strongly suspected that excess accumulation of abdominal fat may help cause diabetes and increase the risk of heart disease. Waist-to-hip ratio (or simple waist circumference) is rapidly becoming a simple and useful tool for gauging the priority that should be attached to weight reduction in different individuals. As there is no way of selectively losing abdominal fat, one should not become too preoccupied with waist-to-hip ratio. Note that abdominal fat seems to be lost more rapidly than other fat during general weight reduction.

Weight cycling or 'yo-yo' dieting

At any one time, a high proportion of the adult population report that they are on a slimming diet (perhaps a third of American women) and yet the proportion who are overweight or obese continues to rise. Even people who are initially successful in losing weight tend to regain it in the following months and years. Many people experience cycles of weight loss and regain, known as weight cycling or '**yo-yo**' **dieting**. Is this weight cycling harmful? If it is, then despite the benefits of weight loss, dieting could do more harm than good.

It does seem to become increasingly difficult for people to lose weight successfully after previous cycles of weight loss and regain. Perhaps the most obvious and likely explanation of this effect is that people become so dispirited by repeated cycles of loss and regain that they find it increasingly difficult to summon up the will to adhere to their latest weight loss programme. However, it has also been suggested that as periods of dieting and weight loss usually lead to loss of lean tissue as well as fat then the net effect of each cycle of weight loss and regain might be to replace some lean tissue with fat, so reducing metabolic rate and making the person more liable to gain weight. Note that the more rapid the weight loss, the greater the loss of lean tissue. It has also been argued that this replacement of lean tissue with fat might predispose yo-yo dieters to diabetes, coronary heart disease and premature death.

In general, studies with experimental animals have not supported this suggestion of a shift in body composition, from lean to fat, and consequent reduction in metabolic rate with repeated cycles of weight loss and regain.

One study attempted to test this directly with a group of obese women. These women went through three cycles of weight loss and regain – two weeks on a very low calorie diet (weight loss) and then four weeks when they were allowed to eat freely (partial weight regain). There was no evidence of any replacement of lean tissue with fat or that metabolic rate fell during the course of this experiment. As expected, resting metabolic rate did fall during the periods of strict dieting, but this rose back to normal when the women were allowed to eat freely. Even in this study, however, the amount of weight loss decreased progressively in the three diet periods probably because compliance with the diet decreased.

Despite such reassurance, there have been several disquieting reports that have found an association between weight fluctuation or instability and increased mortality. The problem is how to interpret these findings. Does weight instability cause increased mortality (cause and effect) or does ill-health and thus increased mortality risk lead to weight instability (effect and cause)? One large American study found that both weight loss and fluctuations in weight were indeed associated with increased mortality. However, the men who had lost weight or whose weight fluctuated also tended to be in poorer health than those whose weight had remained stable. In healthy men who had never smoked, there was no association between either weight loss or weight fluctuation and higher mortality. This suggests that much of the association between weight fluctuation and mortality may be due to the effects of smoking or pre-existing disease and thus that weight cycling *per se* is not a health hazard to healthy non smokers.

Many people manage to achieve substantial temporary weight loss in order to feel and look good at certain important events or periods in their lives, for example, to attend some important social function or when they start a new job. There is no convincing evidence that these bouts of weight loss and regain do them direct physical harm.

The benefits of weight loss

Severe obesity is a substantial health risk and significant health benefits result from even modest weight loss, say 5–10 per cent of initial weight. Weight loss often reduces the symptoms or complications of conditions such as diabetes, hypertension, osteoarthritis and gout which are caused or aggravated by obesity. Risk factors for heart disease and strokes are reduced by weight loss and this may improve future health prospects even in those who are only moderately overweight.

In severely obese people, weight loss improves their self-esteem and social functioning, not least because of improvements in mobility and stamina that result from weight reduction. They have more self-confidence and are less self-conscious about participating in a range of activities that they would not have attempted before, for example, swimming or dancing. Even in those who are only moderately overweight, then, successful weight reduction often gives them a psychological and social boost.

Should I try to lose weight?

Most dieters either fail to lose weight or rapidly regain weight once they stop dieting. So do the potential benefits of weight reduction justify the 'pain' of dieting, the reduction in self-esteem that failure brings, and perhaps even the risk of precipitating a serious eating disorder? Below is a list of some specific groups for whom dieting or weight loss may be undesirable unless under medical advice or supervision:

- In people who are underweight (defined as a BMI of less than 20).
- In people who are not overweight (i.e. BMI less than 25). However, there may be a case for modest weight correction below this threshold if there has been a recent upward drift in weight. The further below 25 the BMI is, then the stronger the case for counselling against weight reduction becomes.
- During pregnancy and lactation – dieting may adversely affect the baby's growth and the quality of milk.
- In older people (say, over 70 years) unless the degree of overweight is substantial and/or there is a medical condition, such as diabetes, that is exacerbated by overweight.
- When someone is acutely ill or injured, unless the condition is exacerbated by overweight.
- In growing children.

Ultimately, the decision about whether or not to embark on a weight reduction programme must be a personal and largely emotional one. All that I can hope to do is to offer some advice that may help to make that decision more rational. Some of the factors that should influence your decision are discussed below.

Your age and sex

The health consequences of excess body weight seem to be greatest in young adults, especially young men. In older people, a little excess weight may actually be advantageous to short- and even medium-term health prospects. The younger you are then the stronger the case for trying to lose weight if you are overweight or obese.

Your waist-to-hip ratio

Fat in the abdomen seems to be more detrimental to health than fat on the limbs and hips. The case for active weight reduction is stronger in those who are overweight (BMI 25–30) if they are apple-shaped, i.e. have a high waist-to-hip ratio.

Your general state of health

The case for specific action to lower body weight would strengthen if you have diabetes, hypertension, gout or if your excess weight is reducing your ability to carry out the tasks of everyday living.

How overweight you are

Finally, and most obviously, the more overweight you are, the stronger is the case for attempting weight loss. If you are severely obese (say BMI over 40), then the potential health and social consequences of your obesity are large and weight loss is medically very desirable. Even modest reductions in weight yield substantial benefits. If your BMI is in the 30–40 range then the health risks and other consequences of your obesity rise sharply over this range and become quite marked once your BMI reaches the high 30s. If your BMI is in the 25–30 range then there may be some negative implications for your long-term health. However, to put these risks in perspective, if you have a lifestyle that is healthy in other respects, for example, you drink in moderation, are a non-smoker, have a good diet and are physically active, then your health prospects are probably better than the average person in the ideal weight range. Some very extensive and persuasive studies conducted in Dallas, Texas by Dr Steven Blair have found that people who are physically fit seem to be protected from many of the consequences of being overweight. Physically fit people who are overweight or even mildly obese seem to live longer and healthier lives than those of ideal weight who are unfit. People in this group should try to ensure that they do not allow their body weight to drift upwards into the 30+ BMI range where the adverse effects start to become more marked.

Of course, many people who diet are not overweight, or only marginally so, and are unlikely to gain health benefits from weight reduction. They are dieting solely for the sake of their appearance, perhaps aiming for some image of body shape that is unreasonable for them and certainly not justified upon health grounds. Perhaps they should consider accepting that their current weight is right for them rather than embarking upon yet another cycle of weight loss and regain. Even if you are slightly overweight, then, this may be a sensible option provided that you are active, fit and eating a healthy low fat diet. Your healthy lifestyle should at least make it much less likely you will get any fatter. But beware! Are you sure that you are as active and eat as healthily as you think? When people are asked to record how much they eat and how much exercise they take then people generally, and obese people especially, tend to under-record their intake and exaggerate their level of activity. Many people mistakenly equate 'busy' with active.

The decision to accept your current weight should be a positive and constructive choice rather than a negative acceptance of defeat. You should try to value yourself as you are, if you see yourself as unattractive and worthless then this opinion will almost certainly be reflected in others. If you transmit a friendly and confident image of yourself, if your body is toned by exercise, if you dress and use make-up wisely then, despite being slightly overweight, you may be pleasantly surprised at the response others give you. Are the images of pencil-thin, skeletal models sometimes seen in the media really most people's (men's) view of what the ideal woman should look like. Of course, these models have been selected for their outstanding natural beauty and photographed in the most flattering way, so even in a state of near emaciation they still look beautiful. This does not mean that most men prefer women to be this shape. The essential difference between a mature woman's body and that of a man are the curves. Whenever film-makers want to portray a stereotype of a female sex symbol then the curvaceousness of the actress or cartoon character is always accentuated. So, why do many women try to starve or exercise these curves out of their bodies?

Pencil-thin models without female curves have been said to reflect the preferences of homosexual men who are reputed to dominate the fashion industry or even that they pander to the latent paedophilic tendencies of some men. Some research has found that men rate women, with small waists in relation to their hips (low waist-to-hip ratio) as attractive. Women with fat stored on their hips are likely to be the ones with better prospects for reproductive success and perhaps men are programmed by evolution to choose these women. Although pin-up models and beauty contest winners have got thinner over the years, others have found that the waist-to-hip ratio of these women has actually remained remarkably constant. Starvation produces flattening of curves rather than the desired hourglass figure.

To sum up

Whether you are obese, overweight or of normal weight, some general changes in health-related behaviours, such as increased activity and a reduced fat diet should improve your health prospects, make further weight gain unlikely and in the long-term may lead to some weight loss. Failure to conform to these dietary and lifestyle patterns are important causes of obesity (see Chapter 4). If widely implemented, these diet and lifestyle changes would prevent many people becoming overweight and would make some contribution to reducing levels of overweight and obesity in the population.

If you are not overweight then adopting these general measures will reduce the risk of you becoming so. Prevention is better than cure, especially where most cures are painful and have very low long-term success rates. Weighing oneself regularly, say twice a month, gives an unequivocal early warning of weight gain and allows one to take action, whilst the amount of excess weight is still relatively small. As the required weight loss grows so the prospect of weight normalisation becomes more daunting; the need to lose large amounts of weight may evoke feelings of despair and helplessness which diminishes the chances of success. Parents should try to instill good dietary habits and encourage their children to be active.

I am not advocating life-long dieting and preoccupation with body weight. When one understands the behaviours that cause weight gain then one can adopt a low risk pattern of living without continually being conscious of the need to count calories. I would specifically counsel against becoming too preoccupied with being thin and against fostering an unhealthy preoccupation with dieting and weight loss in children which could precipitate an eating disorder.

Adopting a healthy lifestyle

An active lifestyle (for all) and a low fat diet (for adults) have substantial benefits for health and wellbeing over and above their effects on body weight. They can thus be promoted in their own right without having to continually focus upon their effects upon body weight. One could argue that much that passes for health promotion or education tends to focus too much upon measured parameters such as blood cholesterol, blood pressure, BMI and even waist-to-hip ratio. We become so fearful of high measurements that changing them becomes an end in its own right, rather than a means to better health prospects. Some treatments that are effective in lowering blood cholesterol or blood pressure may actually increase death rates and so their net effect is a negative one.

If more emphasis was put upon promoting and facilitating behaviours that are beneficial to health, such as taking regular exercise, eating a good diet, moderating alcohol usage and avoiding tobacco, then changes in these measured parameters would inevitably follow. A recent editorial in the *New England Journal of Medicine* (1995) suggested that it might be time to shift the emphasis of research and health education away from body weight *per se* and focus more upon the behaviours that lead to excessive weight gain. We, as consumers, should concentrate more on making healthier food choices and increasing physical activity which should assist in lifetime weight control. Research should focus upon the behavioural and cultural barriers that prevent us adopting this lifestyle pattern.

By themselves, these general measures are unlikely to correct established obesity. If you are obese then you will almost certainly have to take active and painful steps to restrict your calorie intake – you will have to 'go on a diet'. To lose substantial amounts of accumulated fat may require months of serious dieting. Even those who are only overweight may well need to adopt specific and prolonged weight reduction measures if they wish to lose excess weight that has already accumulated, although adopting this healthier lifestyle pattern should at least make it much less likely that you will gain more weight and slip into the more dangerous obese category.

When obesity is severe and intractable, then more aggressive treatments may be considered – anti-obesity drugs; **very low calorie diets (VLCDs)**; or even surgical procedures like having your jaw wired or the capacity of your stomach reduced by surgical stapling. With such treatments, there is always the danger that the cure may be more harmful than the obesity. The likelihood that the risks of weight loss measures will exceed the benefits is increased if these aggressive interventions are used in mild to moderate obesity where the risks from the obesity are smaller. If the weight loss induced by aggressive interventions proves to be only temporary, then this makes it even more difficult to justify their use.

Conclusions

- There are clearly adverse health and social consequences associated with being overweight and particularly with being obese.
- The adverse consequences of obesity are greater in the young and if the fat is concentrated around the abdomen.
- The consequences of being overweight or even mildly obese are relatively small if the person is otherwise healthy and if their diet and lifestyle is healthy, particularly if they are fit and active.
- There is little evidence that being slightly underweight is harmful but being severely underweight, including that associated with eating disorders, does have very serious health consequences.
- There is no convincing evidence that cycles of weight loss and regain are directly harmful.
- Increased activity and a reduction in dietary fat will lessen the risk of gaining excess weight, make a contribution to long-term weight correction and have substantial health benefits in their own right.
- Reasonably rapid or substantial weight loss will probably also require prolonged calorie restriction.

3 | ENERGY BALANCE AND ITS CONTROL

Scope of the chapter

In this chapter, I will discuss the concept of energy balance, the notion that stable weight requires that the intake of calories in food and drink must exactly equal the number of calories used by the body in keeping its systems working and in activity. I will review current scientific theories about how the body regulates energy balance and thus how body weight and fat storage are regulated.

Energy balance – the concept

When we digest and metabolise our food we release its chemical energy so that this energy can be used for body functions, for example, energy for breathing and to keep the heart beating and energy to make our muscles work. This process of 'metabolising' food to generate the energy for body functions is rather like a power station burning coal to convert the chemical energy in the coal into the electrical energy that drives the electrical equipment in our homes and factories.

It is one of the fundamental laws of science that 'energy cannot be created or destroyed, only changed from one form to another'. This means that if a person's weight is stable (i.e. body energy content remains constant), all of the energy available from their food has either been used to keep the body's internal organs working or used to do external work, such as move the body or lift something.

When the energy available from a day's food and drink is equal to the energy expended by the body then we are said to be in **energy balance** (see Figure 3.1). As energy intake exactly equals expenditure then total body energy stores remain stable and so should body weight.

If positive then body
energy stores increase
either due to growth of
lean tissue and/or
increase in fat stores.

⬆

| Energy in (food/drink) | − | Energy out (expended in body functions and activity) | = | The energy balance ➡ If zero then weight is stable. |

⬇

If negative, body
energy stores fall due
to loss of fat and/or
lean.

3.1 The energy balance equation

If the energy available from our food and drink is greater than that which is used during the day then this surplus cannot simply disappear. We have a **positive energy balance** and the surplus energy is stored within the body. In a child, some storage of surplus energy is essential to allow for growth – as the body grows so its energy content increases. Some adults also need a positive energy balance, for example, pregnant women and those recovering after a period of weight loss due to starvation or illness. For other adults, a positive energy balance means that the surplus energy intake is being stored as fat. This stored fat can be used as a reserve energy supply if famine or illness prevent us eating enough. In our power station analogy, if electricity production exceeds current demand then the surplus energy could be stored in some way for future use, for example, by pumping water to an uphill reservoir which can later be used for hydro-electric generation.

If the amount of food energy eaten is less than the amount of energy used then the person is said to have a **negative energy balance**. The deficit is made up from the body's energy stores and so the person loses fat (and lean). When dieting, we strive to achieve a negative energy balance by reducing intake and increasing output (by exercise). If body stores are completely used up, then bodily functions cease and the person dies of starvation. If a power station receives insufficient fuel and there is no 'store' of electricity then power cuts occur.

Control of energy balance – possible strategies

Many adults maintain a stable weight over long periods of their adult lives and so they must be in overall energy balance; any small surpluses on some days are balanced by small deficits on other days. Physiological control mechanisms help to maintain this energy balance. For increasing numbers of people, however, there is not a balance between small energy surpluses and deficits but rather there is a sustained surplus which results in excess fat accumulating. If sustained, then only a tiny imbalance is necessary to explain huge long-term weight gains. For example, in order to gain 20 kg (45 lb) of fat tissue over a ten year period, it would require a daily surplus of only 40 calories, i.e. less than the energy in the butter or margarine we might spread on a piece of bread.

In order to achieve energy balance, *either* the intake of food energy must be controlled so that it matches the energy used, *or* expenditure of energy regulated to match the energy consumed. Some combination of these two strategies is also possible. Returning to our power station analogy, this station might have sensing systems able to monitor the outflow of electrical power, the size of any 'stores' of electricity and the energy value of the coal entering the furnaces. This information would feed into a central computer. The computer could then *either* regulate coal input so that it supplied the present electricity demand and maintained the 'stores' *and/or* control the inflow of cooling water from a river and thus the amount of surplus energy disposed of by warming this water and returning it to the river. This latter option appears wasteful, but it might be necessary if our power station required a minimum fuel-burn to keep it operational. Likewise, there may be good physiological reasons for maintaining a certain minimum intake of food even if the body has ample stores of fat (see later in the chapter).

Is energy expenditure regulated?

We are all aware of energy intake being controlled because we experience the feelings of hunger and satiation (i.e. satisfied or quenched hunger), but does control of energy output play any part in energy balance control?

At one time, it was argued that taking in too much food might increase the urge to take more exercise and burn off more calories. It is certainly true that starving people tend to curtail their activity and conserve energy. However, general experience suggests that gluttony and sloth often go together – a heavy meal is more likely to produce the desire to sleep than to exercise. Any desire to exercise provoked by overeating is more likely to be the result of a guilty conscience than due to some physiological control mechanism – 'I know I've overeaten so I should try to walk it off!'

Another theory suggests that we can burn off surplus calories in 'futile' **thermogenic** (i.e. heat-generating) metabolic pathways. The term **adaptive thermogenesis** (adaptive heat generation), has been used to describe this 'burning off' process.

When people are starving or dieting, their energy use certainly does decrease for the following reasons:

- there is less food to digest, absorb and assimilate – these processes each have an energy cost;
- in severe starvation, physical activity is usually curtailed;
- as the body gets smaller so there is less tissue to maintain and to move;
- there is an increase in metabolic efficiency, perhaps related to changes in body temperature regulation.

This means that during starvation and weight loss, the amount of energy needed to maintain balance declines. As a consequence of this, many dieters find that a diet initially succeeds in achieving weight loss but then their weight sticks and they need to reduce their intake still further to get continued weight loss.

Conversely, when people overeat their rate of energy expenditure increases for the reasons listed below:

- there is more food to digest, absorb and assimilate;
- surplus food calories are converted to fat and this is an energy-requiring process, particularly if the excess calories are in the form of carbohydrate or protein;
- if the body gets bigger, there is more body to maintain and so metabolic rate increases;
- as the body gets bigger, so the energy costs of any movement increase.

The only area of dispute is about whether overfeeding results in some increase in expenditure above and beyond these increases, for example, as a result of some adaptive mechanism whose primary function is to burn off surplus calories and prevent weight gain.

This has been investigated by paying volunteers (often students or prisoners) for deliberately overeating. In some such studies the volunteers stored less fat than would have been expected from their apparent food intake – some surplus calories appeared to have been 'burnt off' by adaptive thermogenesis. Some more recent studies have found little, if any, evidence of this burning off process. In such studies, it is difficult to know how much to allow for the inevitable increases in energy expenditure that must follow overfeeding (listed above) and to be sure that devious subjects have not disposed of some of the food they were paid to eat.

Studies on animals

Several studies with animals have found convincing evidence that, under some conditions, surplus calories can be burnt off, for example, in certain adult rats persuaded to overeat by the provision of a tasty and varied diet. In 1979, it was suggested by Dr Mike Stock and Dr Nancy Rothwell in London that a tissue known as **brown fat** was the principal site of this burning off process (adaptive thermogenesis) at least in rats and mice. Brown fat is a tissue that is known to be capable of generating considerable amounts of heat – small animals use heat generated in brown fat to keep themselves warm in cold weather. The ob/ob mouse is a widely used animal model of obesity. These mice are born with a genetic defect which makes them become very obese. Some studies in the late 1970s seemed to suggest that the severe obesity of these animals might be caused by their inability to generate heat in their brown fat. Ob/ob mice generate less heat than lean mice, they have low body temperatures and die when exposed to the cold. Even if they are only allowed to eat as much as lean mice, they still get much heavier and fatter. Their obesity seemed to be partly the result of reduced heat production that made them use less energy and not just due to overeating.

These brown fat studies generated considerable excitement in the early 1980s. They appeared to offer the prospect of a painless cure for obesity, a drug that would stimulate brown fat and so simply 'burn off' surplus calories. Some nutritionists argued that this 'burning off' process was a major contributor to normal energy balance control in people as well as in rats. It was suggested that differences in people's capacity for adaptive thermogenesis might explain apparent differences in susceptibility to weight gain. Thus, some people might remain lean despite eating a lot by burning off surplus calories whilst other people would fatten easily because they are unable to burn off surplus calories and so have to store more of them as fat.

On reflection, it now seems probable that brown fat and adaptive thermogenesis may have limited relevance to human energy balance regulation. Brown fat has generally been thought of as non-functional or even non-existent in adult human beings (human babies do use it to produce heat because they cannot shiver and are prone to hypothermia). Human adults do not need brown fat because they use other methods to keep warm, for example, putting on more clothes, reducing blood flow to the skin surface, and by generating heat by shivering. New techniques have made it possible to demonstrate unequivocally that obese people have higher rather than lower metabolic rates than lean people (i.e. they generate more heat) and most do not have a defect in their heat generating capacity. Nevertheless, even if there is only a small capacity for adaptive thermogenesis (whether in brown fat or elsewhere) it could still make an important contribution to preventing the tiny positive energy balances that, over decades, result in large amounts of weight gain. Likewise, thermogenic drugs, if safe enough to be used for extended periods, might still make some contribution to weight loss programmes.

Even the reduced heat generation of ob/ob mice may not be the direct result of an inability to generate heat. Starved mice, like starved people, reduce their energy expenditure. One way in which mice do this is to allow their body temperature to fall well below normal for several hours at a time. This condition is called torpor, and it saves energy that the mouse would normally use to keep warm. If the genetic problem of these mice fooled their brain into 'believing' that they had no fat stores then they should respond as if continuously starved, for example, by curtailing their activity, eating more and reducing their heat production to produce a semi-permanent state of torpor. Their low body temperature, inactivity and high food intake could all be the result of their brain being fooled into believing that they are starving and inappropriately initiating energy conserving mechanisms. The recent discovery of leptin (see later in the chapter) seems to confirm this explanation of their low body temperature.

Control of energy intake

'External' influences upon feeding

The power station in our analogy has continuous inflow of a single fuel controlled by a computer that is influenced solely by objective information. People, on the other hand, eat intermittent meals made up of foods of varied composition and energy value. Eating is partly controlled by objective 'internal' physiological signals but it is also a conscious, voluntary act and other so-called 'external' influences also affect our decisions about when, what and how much to eat. These 'external' influences upon eating include:

■ culture and social conventions, such as eating times, are often culturally prescribed and how much we eat may be greatly influenced by others (it may cause offence to leave food);

■ the palatability of food and the pleasure derived from eating;

■ habit, for example, always eating a particular snack when watching a movie;

■ our psychological state, for example, eating to relieve anxiety, boredom or unhappiness.

Perhaps only in newborn babies is human feeding controlled largely by internal physiological mechanisms. Babies demand food when they are hungry. After infancy, we learn to eat in response to other non-physiological, 'external' cues. This may make us less responsive to our internal physiological cues or even cause us to consciously override them.

'Internal' physiological regulation of feeding

After a few hours without food we are aware of the need to eat – **hunger**. This powerful drive can force hungry people to eat bizarre things or do desperate things to obtain food. Once we have eaten, then this hunger drive is quenched or 'satiated'.

The brain systems that control feeding are referred to as the **appestat** (c.f. thermostat) because they are envisaged as controlling food intake to match energy needs in much the same way as a thermostat regulates heat input to control a room's temperature. The **hypothalamus** is an area of the brain that is known to control several body functions such as body temperature, growth and thirst. Reports in the early medical literature of overeating and massive weight gain after damage to the hypothalamus indicated that it was also important in the control of feeding and energy balance. In the early

1940s, technological developments made it possible to destroy or electrically stimulate specific areas deep within the brain. This technique can give useful clues as to the functions of different parts of the brain. Damage to one area, the ventromedial hypothalamus (VMH), caused rats to overeat and become very obese. Damage to another area, the lateral hypothalamus (LH), completely abolished eating (and drinking) behaviour and these animals would starve to death despite food being available. Stimulation of the lateral hypothalamus (LH) could provoke eating in animals and stimulation of the ventromedial hypothalamus (VMH) could temporarily halt food seeking and eating in hungry animals.

In the 1950s, the dual-centre hypothesis of food intake regulation gave a very simple model of how the system for regulating food intake (appestat) might work (see Figure 3.2). It was envisaged that there was a feeding centre in the lateral hypothalamus (LH) which was responsible for evoking hunger and food seeking behaviour. This explained why damage to the LH caused loss of food seeking and eating behaviour and why stimulation of the LH evoked food seeking and eating in rats. In the ventromedial hypothalamus (VMH), a satiety centre was envisaged which would periodically suppress the feeding centre and this would lead to

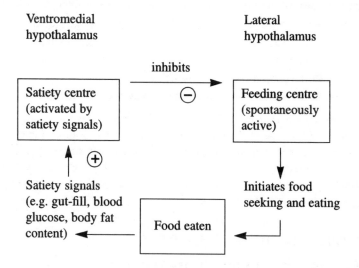

3.2 The dual-centre hypothesis of food intake regulation

satiation. This satiety centre would be activated by certain **satiety signals** that indicated that fat reserves and food intake were adequate. Destruction of this area induced overeating and obesity in experimental animals. Although other areas in the hypothalamus and the rest of the brain are now known also to play a role in regulating feeding, the key importance of the hypothalamus in regulating food intake (and probably energy expenditure) has been confirmed. The ways in which all of these brain areas interconnect and interact to control feeding is still unclear and is beyond the scope of this book.

The dual-centre hypothesis in Figure 3.2 is now regarded as a rather naive oversimplification of the brain mechanisms regulating food intake. Nevertheless, this simple model does have the three basic elements that any system for controlling food intake must have:

- a series of information inputs – satiety signals;
- areas in the brain that integrate this information – the appestat;
- a feeding drive that can be modified in response to the satiety inputs.

In our power station analogy, these correspond respectively to:

- the systems that feed information about fuel flow, the size of any electricity stores and power demand into the central computer;
- the central computer itself;
- the system that adjusts the flow of fuel into the furnace.

Satiety signals transmit information to the brain's appestat about feeding status and the size of the body's energy stores. The ability to manipulate these satiety signals and thus control the hunger drive would be of immense practical value in the treatment of obesity. In the next section we look at some possible satiety signals and the ways in which they may affect hunger and feeding.

Possible satiety signals
(1) Signals originating from the gut

Sensory (i.e. sensing) nerves in the gut, or hormones released from the gut, might relay to the brain information about the volume and composition of food within it.

When we are hungry, then our empty stomach undergoes rhythmic 'hunger contractions' or hunger pangs. These hunger pangs are controlled by the 'unconscious' part of our nervous system and they are one of the uncomfortable sensations that we interpret as hunger. We therefore eat in order to relieve this discomfort. These hunger pangs may even produce audible rumbling sounds that notify others of our hunger! When we have eaten a large meal, then we are aware of the stretching of our stomachs. This full feeling is initially reassuring and pleasurable but if we continue to eat then it becomes uncomfortable and dissuades us from further eating. These experiences suggest that signals from the gut do normally play some role in the control of feeding.

Meals usually end well before much absorption has occurred and certainly before there have been changes in the size of the body energy stores. This strongly suggests that signals arising directly from the gut play some role in signalling the end of a meal. The intake of food will activate stretch sensors in the gut and these will feed information to the brain via sensing nerves. Eating causes the release of hormones from the gut and these may also affect the appestat in the brain. For example, the hormone cholecystokinin (CCK) is released from the intestine when food is present and it reduces hunger and inhibits feeding by activating sensing nerves in the gut that relay information to the appestat.

The **energy density** of a diet is its energy concentration – the number of calories obtained from a given amount of food. One can produce rat diets with widely varying energy densities by adding either fat (energy concentrated) or a bulking agent like methyl cellulose (adds bulk but no calories). These changes in energy concentration would be expected to interfere with any system for controlling food intake that relied upon sensing food volume. When rats are fed a very concentrated diet, this should reduce satiety signals from the gut; nevertheless the rats reduce the amount of food they eat although not by enough to compensate for its higher energy content and so they tend to gain weight. High fat, energy dense diets have been used as one way of producing experimental obesity in rats. If the rat's diet is made very bulky this should increase satiety signals from the gut. However, the rats compensate quite effectively for this energy dilution and eat enough of the dilute food to satisfy their calorie needs.

Signals caused by the presence of food in the gut do play some role in signalling satiation. However, these signals can be overridden by other signals, particularly if they indicate body energy deprivation – even cutting all the sensing nerves from a rat's stomach does not prevent the rat from maintaining some control of its food intake and body weight. Rats fed very dilute diets compensate by eating more of this food because information from other sensors indicates that the animal is energy deficient. When food is very concentrated, then, despite some reduction in the amount the animal eats, the animal tends to take in too many calories and gains weight even though other satiety signals should register the oversupply of energy. The system appears to be better at preventing undersupply of energy than oversupply.

(2) Blood levels of digested food components

After eating, the rise in blood levels of amino acids (from digested protein) and glucose (from digested carbohydrate) could act as satiety signals. An average meal might take four hours to digest and absorb, so if we eat the standard three meals per day, then for most of our waking hours we are absorbing food (and food is present in the gut). Only in the pre-lunch and pre-dinner periods and during the night, are we in the so-called post absorptive state – nothing is being digested or absorbed from the gut.

The satiety effects of blood glucose concentration have been particularly well studied. After eating a meal that contains carbohydrate (as most meals do), then blood glucose concentration rises as this carbohydrate is digested and absorbed. The rise in blood glucose concentration triggers the release of the hormone **insulin** from the pancreas. Insulin increases the uptake and metabolism of glucose by the tissues. In general, high blood glucose and insulin concentrations, and high rates of glucose metabolism, occur after feeding and are associated with satiation. During fasting, blood glucose and insulin concentrations are low and use of glucose in metabolism is low because many tissues are switched over to using fat during fasting – such conditions are associated with hunger. These observations led to the suggestion that blood glucose concentration or the rate of glucose metabolism might regulate feeding – the **glucostat theory**.

Early versions of the 'glucostat' theory envisaged glucose-sensing cells in the appestat that monitored blood glucose concentration. After a meal, when blood glucose was high, then these glucose sensors were activated and produced satiation. When glucose levels fell during fasting, then hunger was restored. When gold thioglucose (effectively glucose molecules with gold attached to them) was injected into mice, the gold accumulated in the ventromedial hypothalamus causing irreparable damage to the nerve cells and leading to permanent obesity in the mice. This provided persuasive support for the notion that glucose 'sensor' molecules were abundant in this area and it was they that caused the gold (attached to glucose) to selectively accumulate and kill the nerve cells.

In untreated diabetes, one may get ravenous hunger despite high blood glucose concentrations which seems inconsistent with this idea that high blood glucose produces satiation. However, the blood glucose concentration of diabetics is high because they lack the insulin which allows glucose to get into many cells and so it just accumulates in the blood because it is unable to be used. As cells cannot take up glucose, they are deprived of glucose despite the high blood concentration. In diabetes, glucose metabolism is low and fat utilisation high because glucose is not getting into the cells to allow it to be used. During fasting, glucose use is also low but in this case it is because there is a low glucose supply due to the low concentration in the blood. It has therefore been suggested that a high rate of glucose use in metabolism may cause satiation rather than high blood concentration. When the rate of glucose metabolism is high (and therefore use of fat low) then this results in satiation. In healthy people, this occurs after eating carbohydrate. When glucose metabolism is low (and therefore that of fat is high) this results in hunger. This occurs during fasting, in untreated diabetes and if meals with little or no carbohydrate are eaten. Insulin is normally released when carbohydrate is eaten and allows glucose to be taken up and metabolised by the cells and this leads to satiation. (Note that large doses of injected insulin cause blood glucose to fall sharply and produce hunger.)

The products of carbohydrate digestion are involved in satiation and they probably act via several different routes. For example, as well as any direct effects of glucose on cells in the appestat, sensing nerves in the liver relay information to the appestat about the relative rates of glucose and fat use by liver cells.

Use of fat in metabolism is associated with hunger. Carbohydrate intake increases use of carbohydrate and reduces use of fat, but fat intake has little effect on either fat or carbohydrate metabolism. As fat is absorbed, much of it is shunted directly into our fat stores – one reason why high fat diets may be less satiating than high carbohydrate diets and seem to predispose to weight gain and obesity.

(3) The size of the body's fat stores

One problem with the satiety signals discussed so far is that it is difficult to see how short-term indicators like stomach fullness or blood glucose concentration could produce accurate long-term regulation of body weight. Accurate control of body weight is easier to explain if one envisages that there is some satiety signal that directly indicates to the appestat the size of the body fat stores. If our power station computer is to control accurately the amount of electrical energy 'stored' as the uphill reservoir of water, then the programming of the computer would be much easier if it was receiving direct information about the size of this store.

In the 1950s, the so-called **lipostat theory** of feeding control was formulated. It was proposed that fat tissue released a 'satiety hormone', now called **leptin**, which acted upon the appestat to reduce hunger. The size of body fat stores determines the amount of leptin released and so controls feeding. Small increases in the amount of stored fat increases the amount of leptin released and so reduces hunger and food intake. If body fat stores become depleted (for example, after fasting) then the depleted fat tissue releases less leptin, leading to increased hunger and increased food intake. Obesity would occur if fat tissue produced too little leptin or if the appestat failed to respond adequately to leptin. For example, damage to the ventromedial hypothalamus in rats produces obesity because it damages the area of the brain where leptin acts to inhibit feeding.

One might expect that such a mechanism would produce a body weight that oscillates around an average value or **'set point'** much as a thermostat causes room temperature to oscillate around the selected 'set point'. If volunteers are weighed every day for a few months then weight does indeed appear to oscillate around a set point. During periods of feasting or illness it may deviate further but still tends to return to the 'set point'. Unfortunately, over a time-scale of years and decades, the apparent set point of our lipostat or fat controller seems to drift slowly upwards in many (most!) Britons and Americans and this slow upward drift, when sustained over several decades, leads to obesity.

Obese (**ob/ob**) and *diabetes* (**db/db**) are two forms of genetic obesity in mice. Both ob/ob and db/db mice inherit a very severe obesity associated with diabetes. Both conditions are due to just one of the animal's proteins being abnormal. In the 1970s, it was proposed that the ob/ob mouse is unable to produce leptin and so its appestat is unable to detect any fat stores and so the animal overeats and gets very fat. It was suggested that in the db/db mouse, the abnormal protein is one that allows the appestat to respond to leptin – because these animals are so fat, they produce leptin in large amounts but their appestat cannot detect the leptin and so once again they cannot sense any fat stores and so they overeat. At this time, leptin had not been discovered and was a purely hypothetical hormone. These suggestions were the result of an ingenious series of parabiosis experiments; these are experiments where pairs of animals are surgically linked together so that hormones and other substances can pass between their blood. The results obtained from four of these parabiotic pairings are explained below.

■ **Pairing**   A normal animal paired with one which has had its ventromedial hypothalamus destroyed.

Result   The animal with the damaged hypothalamus overeats and gains weight as expected. The normal animal eats less and loses weight.

Explanation   The animal with the damaged hypothalamus gets fat as it cannot respond to leptin, but as it gets fatter so its fat cells produce large amounts of leptin. This extra leptin enters the blood of the normal animal and so this animal's appestat 'believes' it is very fat.

■ **Pairing**   A normal and an ob/ob mouse.

Result   The ob/ob mouse eats less and loses weight.

Explanation   The ob/ob mouse is unable to produce its own leptin but can respond to leptin produced by its lean partner and so eats less and loses weight.

■ **Pairing**   A normal and a db/db mouse

Result   The normal mouse stops eating and starves.

Explanation   The db/db mouse cannot respond to leptin and so gets fat and produces excess leptin. This leptin enters the blood of the normal mouse and suppresses feeding – this animal's appestat 'believes' it has massive fat stores.

■ **Pairing**   An ob/ob and a db/db mouse.

Result   The ob/ob mouse eats less and loses weight.

Explanation   The ob/ob mouse is responding to the excess leptin produced by its db/db partner.

This lipostat theory had remained on the 'scientific backburner' for many years; leptin had never been identified and there was only indirect evidence that it actually existed. However, in 1994 a research group in America identified the obese gene and the protein produced from it in healthy mice. This protein is produced exclusively in fat cells and seems to have all of the characteristics expected of the satiety hormone or leptin. In normal lean mice, production of this leptin increases as the amount of fat in the fat cells increases but declines during starvation. Ob/ob mice have a defective leptin gene and so do not produce any active leptin but when leptin is injected into ob/ob mice, they eat less and lose weight; leptin also decreases food intake in normal animals. To sum up, the obese gene produces a protein (leptin) that keeps normal mice (and people) lean. In ob/ob mice this gene is damaged and so functional leptin cannot be produced from it. Note that genes are the body's codes for its proteins – an abnormal gene means that the protein produced from it will not function properly.

Human fat cells also produce a human version of leptin. In 1997 two British children, cousins of Pakistani origin, were found to have mutations in their leptin genes. These children were extremely obese – at the age of eight the girl weighed almost three times the average for her age (86 kg/190 lbs) and at the age of two, the boy weighed two-and-a-half times the average for his age (29 kg/63 lb). These children are the human equivalent of ob/ob mice and their discovery shows directly that leptin deficiency has similar consequences in humans and mice.

Leptin sensors have been found in the ventromedial hypothalamus of mice which indicates that leptin acts here. Leptin does not cause weight loss in db/db mice and this is consistent with earlier suggestions that they become obese because they are unable to respond to leptin. It seems that in db/db mice the genetically defective protein is one that normally enables the appestat to respond to leptin.

These leptin discoveries have been widely reported in the popular press. It has been suggested that in the not too distant future, leptin might offer a simple and effective treatment for obesity (see Chapter 7). Some of this early excitement was tempered by the failure, until mid-1997, to find any leptin deficiency syndrome in obese people; leptin levels are actually higher in obese people than lean people. Most human obesity is unlikely to be caused by leptin deficiency but could be the result of a reduced response to leptin.

Why so many satiety signals?

The apparent multiplicity of satiety inputs to the brain's appestat may seem like a particularly cumbersome system for controlling the size of our fat stores and, given the prevalence of obesity, a rather ineffective one at that. However, controlling body fat levels might be just one function of these mechanisms. One obvious necessity would be to limit meal size and prevent overloading and damage to the gut and perhaps also overloading of the metabolic systems that handle absorbed nutrients. Another function would be to maintain an adequate inflow of energy and essential nutrients. Even if fat stores are excessive, then maintaining a hunger drive and some inflow of food might still be desirable. Most obviously, complete abstinence would deplete the body's stores of some essential nutrients but it would also deprive our tissues and especially our brain of glucose because our glucose stores are very small. During fasting, body protein (lean tissue) is broken down and converted to glucose by an inefficient process that depletes our muscles and essential organs. As we adapt to fasting, fat is converted to **ketones** which can be used by the brain as an alternative to glucose but reliance on ketones may lead to suboptimal functioning and so is something our physiological mechanisms avoid if possible.

Excess fat stores impair our mobility and have detrimental effects on our health. In the industrialised countries, preventing this excess might be considered a priority function of our control systems. However, during most of our evolution the overriding priority shaping our physiology would have been to obtain enough food to ensure that there were sufficient fat stores to survive the inevitable times of famine.

Practical implications for weight control

(1)   If signals from the gut help to control food intake then eating a concentrated diet would decrease these signals and might encourage overconsumption. Fat increases the energy concentration of the diet but starchy foods (potatoes and cereals) and those high in water and fibre (fruits and vegetables) have a relatively low energy concentration.

(2)   If high levels of absorbed nutrients in blood suppress appetite, then the slower a meal is digested and absorbed, the longer these levels are elevated and the longer the satiating effect of the meal should last. Slow digestion and absorption would also prolong any satiety signals due to the

presence of food in the gut. Slowly digested food should have more 'staying power' in its satiating effects. Unrefined foods that are high in starch and fibre seem to produce this 'slow release' effect by delaying stomach emptying and slowing gut absorption. Highly refined foods are digested and absorbed very quickly and lead to rapid but short-lived rises in blood glucose concentration. They may even cause such large and rapid release of insulin that blood glucose falls very rapidly and 'overshoots' the normal level – this rebound **hypoglycaemia** (low blood glucose) may make us feel very hungry shortly after eating. Foods that are high in starch and fibre seem to produce the most sustained satiating effect for a given number of calories.

(3) Carbohydrate intake causes all of the following:

- ■ a rise in blood glucose concentration;
- ■ insulin release;
- ■ increased glucose metabolism;
- ■ decreased fat metabolism.

All of these conditions are associated with absence of hunger. Fat has little effect on any of these parameters and so a given number of carbohydrate calories should have a greater satiating effect than the same number of calories taken as fat. This points towards high carbohydrate, low fat diets for weight loss and weight maintenance.

(4) Leptin injections cure the obesity of ob/ob mice which is caused by leptin deficiency. Leptin also reduces eating and causes some weight loss in lean mice. Leptin deficiency is not a major cause of human obesity and levels are actually high in most obese people. Leptin injections in obese people would not mean a straight replacement of a missing hormone as it does in the ob/ob mouse. Obese people may be unresponsive to leptin (as in the db/db mouse) or they may have become desensitised to leptin by prolonged overeating. The high leptin levels in obese people may not even reflect a decreased physiological response but may rather reflect the fact that external social, cultural and psychological factors persuade us to overeat and partly ignore our internal control mechanisms even when they are functioning normally. These suggestions may make the potential benefits of leptin therapy seem less promising. Nevertheless, leptin may still become an important tool in obesity therapy. It may be especially useful in reducing hunger and thus easing the discomfort of initial weight loss programmes (see Chapter 7).

(5) What about adaptive thermogenesis? Could thermogenic drugs enable people to eat excessively and yet still lose weight because the drug stimulates mechanisms that 'burn off' the surplus calories? Whilst thermogenic drugs are being tested (see Chapter 7), it seems unlikely that in the near future any drug will be able to safely produce large and long-term increases in our energy expenditure. Even the existence of specific mechanisms for 'burning off' surplus calories is still disputed. Note that leptin increases energy expenditure as well as decreasing food intake. The leptin deficiency of ob/ob mice results in reduced energy expenditure as well as increased intake of food.

(6) Exercise certainly does increase energy expenditure and so food intake is not the only controllable variable in the energy balance equation. Inactivity is undoubtedly a major factor predisposing us to obesity (see Chapter 4). Increased activity should reduce our susceptibility to excessive weight gain.

(7) The composition of the diet may also affect energy expenditure. If surplus calories are taken as fat then the energy costs of fat synthesis are much less than if surplus calories are in the form of carbohydrate or protein. On a high fat diet, more surplus calories will be stored as body fat than on a high carbohydrate diet – one more pointer to the use of low fat, high carbohydrate diets for weight control.

(8) Nerve cells transmit messages to each other by means of chemicals that act as messengers or **nerve transmitters**. We are now starting to identify the chemical messengers that nerve cells of the brain's appestat use to communicate with each other. Drugs that block or mimic the actions of these transmitters may be useful in the treatment of obesity (see Chapter 7).

Conclusions

- ■ If body weight is to remain stable then the energy content of food must equal the energy expended by the body.
- ■ If energy intake exceeds expenditure then weight gain occurs either through increased amounts of lean tissue (growth), increased amounts of stored fat, or both.
- ■ If energy expenditure exceeds intake then weight loss must occur.

- To control energy balance and thus body weight, then either the intake of energy, energy expenditure or both must be regulated.

- Areas of the brain known as the appestat regulate energy intake by controlling the hunger drive and probably also control energy expenditure.

- The appestat responds to signals that indicate the feeding state of the person and the size of body fat stores. These are called satiety signals.

- Probable satiety signals are things that indicate: the nature and amount of food in the gut; the blood concentration of food digestion products like glucose; and the amount of fat stored in our fatty tissue.

- Current understanding of hunger control mechanisms suggests that dietary fat is likely to be less satiating than carbohydrate and thus that a high fat diet might lessen the effectiveness of our control systems.

- The existence of mechanisms to burn off surplus calories, adaptive thermogenesis, is still controversial. At present, the only practical way of significantly increasing energy expenditure is by taking more exercise.

4 WHY DO SO MANY OF US GET FAT?

Scope of the chapter

In this chapter, I will try to suggest reasons why affluent industrialised populations are so prone to excessive weight gain, i.e. to suggest causes for the epidemic of obesity that is sweeping across the industrialised world. I will discuss how our increasing understanding of the causes of excessive weight gain might help in controlling this problem.

Survival of the fattest?

'Survival of the fittest' is a key tenet of the theory of evolution. Evolution should produce animals that are well adapted to their environment. So why do so many affluent people seem to be so poorly adapted to their current environment? They store more fat than is good for their health and mobility and even their chances of reproducing. Why has evolution produced such an apparently ineffective system for controlling human body weight?

In the last chapter, I suggested that preventing excess fat accumulation might be just one of the functions of the mechanisms controlling food intake and that traditionally this was probably a low priority function. For most of human existence, and that of our pre-human ancestors, the survival priority would have been to obtain enough food, and to build up sufficient fat stores to cope with frequent, inevitable and possibly prolonged periods of food shortage. An assured food supply and a sedentary way of life are comparatively recent phenomena and still only apply to a favoured sector of the world population. Few members of primitive societies would have had the opportunity to become obese and this is still true in many societies today. The struggle to obtain sufficient food and maintain adequate fat reserves would have been a major selection pressure shaping our physiology. Those best equipped to obtain sufficient food and cope with periods of food shortage would be more likely to survive and reproduce whilst those best equipped for conditions of continual plenty would be 'selected out' during times of famine. We should not be surprised that control systems, of which the evolutionary priority was to prevent deficiency, are rather inefficient at preventing obesity when food is abundant and demand for activity is minimal.

For hunter-gatherers and peasant farmers, getting and preparing food involves considerable physical effort. Prolonged periods of food scarcity are highly probable whilst at other times there may be gluts of food. Substantial stores of fat, accumulated during times of plenty, would help people to survive the periods of famine. There would be little need to prevent excess fat storage because, under these conditions, weight gain would be largely self-limiting because:

■ weight gain and overeating increases energy consumption;
■ primitive diets may limit the tendency/capacity to overeat.

How does overeating increase energy consumption?

It costs energy to eat, digest and absorb extra food and it costs energy to convert any surplus calories into stored fat. If one eats a slice of bread more than one needs, then some of the excess calories will be 'wasted' in their conversion to body fat. Conversion of carbohydrate or protein to fat is more wasteful than converting dietary fat to body fat. Traditional diets tend to be very high in carbohydrate and low in fat, so less of any surplus calories end up as stored fat.

As the body gets bigger, so more food is required to compensate for the energy used by the extra tissue. Obese people have more lean tissue as well as more fat tissue. Even extra fat tissue uses some energy. As people get heavier, they need to eat more to simply maintain their bodies – this would tend to limit excessive weight gain where food supplies are limited.

The energy costs of exercise increase as the body gets heavier. Not only is there more body to move but the energy efficiency of movement also decreases if fat stores are excessive. If activity level is unchanged, one needs to eat more to support this activity. Inactivity is not an option for most peasant farmers or hunter-gatherers – people who don't work, don't eat. In affluent societies, most people are able to reduce their activity; social conditions may even encourage inactivity. Obesity makes activity more stressful, so weight gain encourages inactivity and this limits any rise in energy expenditure.

New sophisticated techniques have allowed scientists for the first time to measure accurately the energy used by free-living people. These studies confirm that obese people do indeed expend more energy than lean people do. The energy expenditure at rest and performing set activities is unquestionably higher in the obese and their total energy expenditure also tends to be higher despite their inactivity.

Obesity impairs speed and agility and could reduce the ability to obtain food. Overweight hunters, whether people or wild animals, are disadvantaged in the competition for food. Even in affluent countries, obesity may reduce earning potential but this is more likely to encourage the consumption of a cheaper and more fattening diet than to restrict energy intake.

How could primitive diets limit the tendency to overeat?

If obtaining food is an arduous activity, then this discourages food seeking and eating that is not driven by hunger. If food is plentiful, palatable and varied then this might encourage eating for pleasure even in the absence of hunger. A predator may wait for days after a kill before it is driven by hunger to hunt again but, if offered some appealing morsel, it might be persuaded to eat before hunger would have driven it to hunt again. Dogs are the descendants of predatory wolves, and are always ready to accept tasty titbits. The fatness of domestic dogs often mirrors that of their human family.

Primitive diets are usually low in fat but high in starch and fibre. During industrialisation, starchy cereals and roots were replaced in part by foods that were rich in fat and sugar. For example, in 1875, starchy foods provided 55 per cent of the calories in the US diet but by 1975 this had dropped to under 20 per cent. Fat calories are probably less satiating than carbohydrate calories and so a starchy diet would discourage overeating. Traditional low fat diets have a low energy concentration, i.e. they are bulky. This would probably limit the capacity of peasant farmers and hunter-gatherers to overeat. The list below illustrates the wide variation in the amount of different foods needed to provide 1000 calories. This list shows that diets which are heavily dependent upon starchy foods (cereals and potatoes) supplemented by fruits, vegetables and some lean meat and fish would be bulky. One needs to eat many pounds of most fruits and vegetables to get 1000 calories and two or three pounds of most starchy staples. Even lean meat and white fish are relatively low in calories. Many modern foods are energy dense and modern methods of preparing and processing foods tend to remove water and fibre but add fat and sugar and so greatly increase their energy concentration.

Food	Weight in grams	Food	Weight in grams
Fruits			
orange	5950	strawberries	
apple	4690	(canned in syrup)	1538
banana	2280	dried dates	370
grapes	1667	fruit pie	
raisins	368	(individual purchased)	271
strawberries	3704		
Vegetables			
lettuce	7143	soya beans (boiled)	709
tomato	5882	tofu (fried)	383
green beans	4000	chick peas (boiled)	836
broccoli	4167	hummus	535
swede (boiled)	9091	lentils (boiled)	1000
red kidney beans			
(boiled)	971		
Starchy staples and products			
potato (boiled)	1389	corn kernels	671
potato (mashed)	962	corn grits	
French fries		(made with water)	1666
(burger outlet)	357	Cornflakes	278
potato crisps (chips)	183	Weetabix	279
yam (boiled)	752	chocolate biscuits	
sweet potato (boiled)	1190	(cookies)	191
rice (boiled)	725	fruit cake	282
spaghetti (boiled)	962	doughnuts (ring)	252

wheat bread	464	pizza	
tortilla/chapatti		(cheese and tomato)	400
(no fat added)	478	quiche	318
porridge			
(made with water)	2041		
(made with whole milk)	862		

Dairy foods

whole milk	1515	Cheddar cheese	243
skimmed milk	3030	butter	136
double cream	223		

Meat, fish and poultry

egg (boiled)	680	sausage roll	210
egg (fried)	560	steak and kidney pie	310
roast turkey meat	714	pork sausage (grilled)	314
roast chicken meat	606	cod (poached)	1064
southern fried chicken	350	cod (fried in batter)	503
chicken nuggets	338	salmon (steamed)	508
grilled rump steak		prawns (boiled)	935
(with fat)	459	fish fingers (fried)	429
(trimmed)	595	fried scampi	
cheeseburger	380	(breaded)	316
salami	204		

Nuts, seeds and oils

peanuts (raw)	177	margarine	136
walnuts	145	low fat spread	256
sunflower seeds	167	vegetable oils	112

Miscellaneous

sugar	254	chocolate	189

Under some circumstances, extreme energy dilution of the diet can limit energy intake by so much that it causes malnutrition. For example, some traditional weaning diets in developing countries have such low energy concentrations that, even under ideal feeding conditions, the child cannot eat enough of the dilute food to meet their energy needs and so the child starves despite being fed as much as they can eat. This starvation is worsened if the child is only fed infrequently, has a poor appetite, frequent bouts of illness etc. As another example of this **energy density** effect, strictly vegetarian (vegan) children tend to be a little lighter and shorter than non-vegetarian children. Vegan diets tend to have low energy density, largely because they are often low in fat and this may limit the calorie intake of vegan children and so limit their growth. The low fat content and energy density of vegetarian and vegan diets is often hailed as one of their advantages for weight conscious adults – Caucasian vegans and vegetarians in the UK, on average, have lower energy intakes and are lighter and leaner than omnivores.

The high energy concentration of affluent diets coupled with a sedentary lifestyle means that we need to eat much less food (in terms of weight) than our hunter-gatherer ancestors. This makes it much easier for us to overeat and become obese.

To sum up

If someone is consuming surplus calories, then their energy expenditure rises as they gain weight and this tends to limit weight gain. This does not apply if they compensate by reducing their activity or increasing their food intake, and in affluent societies most people are able to do either or both of these. Amongst our ancestors, and in peasant societies today, the opportunity to take either of these options would have been limited. The nature of our ancestors' diets, for example their low energy density and relative monotony, discouraged excess calorie intake.

Nature or nurture?

Do people get fat largely because they inherit genes which make them fat or largely because of their diet and way of life? Is obesity a genetic disease that needs a medical cure or a social disease caused by an unhealthy lifestyle? Certain groups and families seem to be very prone to obesity – pointing towards a strong genetic component to their condition. On the other hand, obesity is rare in peasant communities where frugal food supplies and hard physical work are the norm, but is prevalent in places where people are inactive and where food is varied and plentiful – certain circumstances are required for its development.

It's all the fault of my genes!

The most sympathetic view of the obese is that some inherited defect in their physiology has made them highly susceptible to weight gain when circumstances favour it, such as affluence. Obese people are seen as victims of their physiology. Such a view also encourages the belief that behaviour change is unlikely to be effective in the treatment of obesity and that a medical cure for the genetic defect will be required. This absolves the obese person of responsibility for their condition and its correction.

Several genetic causes for human obesity have enjoyed transient popularity, such as:

■ inadequate leptin production or leptin detection, as in some genetically obese mice (see Chapter 3);

■ some defect in the brain's appestat which controls feeding;

■ impaired adaptive thermogenesis i.e. reduced ability to burn off surplus calories.

Evidence for genetic cause(s) of obesity

The use of simple animal models of obesity has encouraged belief in specific physiological causes for human obesity. If single defective genes or damage to the small areas of the brain can provoke obesity in rodents then they might also be the cause of 'real' obesity in people. If the genetic cause(s) of obesity could be found then it should be possible to devise a cure. Discovery of such a cure offers the prospect of immense fame and fortune to its discoverers. For example, millions of dollars were paid for the patent on the leptin gene even though there is no evidence that leptin deficiency is a major cause of human obesity, and even though leptin had no proven therapeutic value (leptin levels are already high in most obese people).

The evidence that inheritance can have a substantial influence upon body fatness is overwhelming. Single genetic mutations in animals, and occasionally in people, can produce extreme obesity and this obesity is very difficult to correct by dietary means. Even in normal animals, fatness is partly heritable and so by selective breeding farmers have been able to substantially alter the proportions of fat and lean in their carcasses.

Some human populations seem to be extremely prone to obesity and have rates of obesity that dwarf even those seen in the USA and the UK. For example, amongst the Polynesian people of Western Samoa and the Pima indians of southern Arizona, the majority of the adult population are obese (BMI over 30). In urban areas of Western Samoa, 60 per cent of men and

75 per cent of women are obese and less than 10 per cent are not overweight (i.e. BMI below 25).

Many populations that have recently become industrialised seem particularly prone to obesity (and diabetes). They have only recently abandoned their traditional lifestyle with its requirement for hard physical work and its limited food supply. Often such populations, such as that of Western Samoa, have a long history of alternating conditions of feast and famine. These populations may have evolved with a set of thrifty genes that make them better able to survive on limited food supplies and to gain weight rapidly when food is plentiful. Industrialisation changes the prevailing social conditions: mechanised transport and sedentary jobs reduce the need for activity; food supplies become assured and plentiful; the variety of food increases; and, the traditional starchy, fibre-rich and bulky diet is replaced with one which is more palatable, more energy concentrated and higher in fat. Their thrifty genes will now merely predispose them to obesity.

In the industrialised countries, obesity (and leanness) does tend to run in families, but how much of this is down to genetics and how much due to their shared diets and lifestyles? Scandinavian studies that have looked at the fatness levels of twins and of adopted children seem to suggest that genetics is largely responsible for these family trends. For example:

- ■ Fatness levels are more similar in genetically identical twins than in non-identical twins. When twins share the same environment then the fatness levels in identical twins are closer because they share more common genes.
- ■ When identical twins are adopted and reared apart, their levels of fatness still tend to be similar. Despite their differing environments, their common genes mean that the fatness levels in these separated twins are still similar.
- ■ Large surveys of adopted children in Denmark have found that the BMI of adopted children and their natural relatives (parents and siblings) still tend to be similar and almost as similar as those in natural families. Even when family members have different environments, their common genes mean that their fatness levels tend to be similar.

Of course, the diet and lifestyle of people within Scandinavian society may be relatively homogeneous, and the differences between the genetic and adopted families may be relatively small. This would tend to exaggerate the influence of genetics and give the false impression that we are all totally the prisoners of our genes when it comes to fatness.

Obesity is due to gluttony and sloth

A harsher and more judgemental view of obesity has traditionally prevailed – the belief that it is caused by gluttony and sloth. The following quotations from textbooks of the 1930s and 1940s illustrate this view:

> '...99% of cases [of obesity] are due to wrong eating or lack of exercise.'

> 'Obesity in adults is often a result of over indulgence in food and of sedentary habits and should not be explained and excused by pronouncing the persons victims of glandular deficiencies.'

> 'The result of excessive calorie intake or, in other words greed, is obesity.'

> '...abnormality in weight is due to dietary indiscretion.'

Obese people are often regarded as largely to blame for their own condition because they are self-indulgent, lack the willpower to control their appetites and perhaps overeat to compensate for their emotional problems. One 1979 survey found that even amongst professionals treating obesity, it was widely regarded as a self-inflicted condition caused by overeating, that was triggered by emotional problems in people who were weak and self-indulgent. These views would undoubtedly fuel the derision and discrimination experienced by obese people.

Treatment seems simple, the obese person must learn, or be taught, to control their appetites and their laziness. However, treatment is likely to fail because obese people do not have the strength of character or emotional stability to succeed. Whatever the causes of obesity are, these views seem unreasonably harsh because there is no evidence of high levels of psychological or emotional problems in obese people (see Chapter 2) and secondly, because only a tiny, long-term energy imbalance is necessary to produce massive obesity (see Chapter 3).

Evidence that behaviour and diet are the cause(s) of obesity

There is also plenty of evidence to show that environmental influences are important in causing obesity. Farmers can alter the proportions of fat and lean in their animals' carcasses by manipulating their diet as well as by selective breeding. In laboratory animals, several 'environmental manipulations' increase fatness, for example, restricting activity; increasing the fat content of their diets; and '**cafeteria feeding**'.

This cafeteria feeding seems to mimic the circumstances of affluent human populations. Rats are offered a variety of tasty and often high fat foods, in addition to their normal pellet food - foods like cookies, cooked meats, chocolate and crisps. When rats are provided with a variety of energy-rich and tasty human foods with little opportunity for exercise then, like people, they often get fat. This obesity has unquestionably been caused by dietary change, although rats do vary genetically in their susceptibility to this obesity.

Even in those human populations that seem to be genetically prone to obesity, it only becomes widespread if certain lifestyle conditions prevail, for example:

- food is plentiful, varied and palatable;
- the diet is high in fat and/or energy dense;
- there is little requirement for physical activity.

Although Polynesian people have long been noted for their large physiques, obesity rates in Western Samoa has spiralled dramatically upwards in recent years. Between 1978 and 1991 rates of obesity increased sharply in all areas of Western Samoa and the increase was particularly dramatic in the rural areas. Until recently, obesity rates were much lower in the rural areas where people were more likely to maintain an active lifestyle and a more traditional diet. This gap has now narrowed as sedentary habits and consumption of imported western food have spread beyond the cities into the rural areas. Even though the people of Western Samoa may be genetically prone to obesity, it is changes in diet and lifestyle that are responsible for the recent massive increases in obesity prevalence.

Studies on the Pima indians provide even more striking evidence of the need for environmental triggers to produce widespread obesity. Several centuries ago, one group of Pima indians settled in southern Arizona whilst another group settled in the mountains of Mexico. These two groups remain genetically very similar. Present day Mexican Pimas do not suffer from widespread obesity, they are subsistence farmers who spend many hours each week in hard physical labour and still eat a fairly traditional low fat, high carbohydrate diet. In contrast, the Arizona Pimas have ceased to be subsistence farmers. They are now a sedentary population who eat a typical high fat American diet and, as a consequence, have one of the highest rates of obesity in the world.

In the industrialised countries, obesity is more common amongst those in the lower social classes. It seems highly improbable that these class differences in obesity prevalence are genetically determined. Recent increases in rates of obesity must be the result of dietary and lifestyle changes – a doubling in ten years of the number of British men who are obese cannot be due to genetic changes. People with similar genetic backgrounds living in different industrialised countries have very different levels of obesity. For example, descendants of immigrants to the United States tend to be fatter than people in their country of origin. Rapid changes in disease rates upon migration is a classical indicator of an environmental cause.

To sum up

There is undoubtedly genetic variability in the susceptibility of people to obesity – only the magnitude of this variability is in doubt. Some individuals and some ethnic groups seem very prone to obesity. There may be some groups and some individuals within all groups whose 'thrifty' genes make it exceedingly difficult for them to remain lean when food is abundant and there is little need for physical labour. Genetic factors may be particularly important in determining which people within our countries become obese.

Despite this, environmental factors seem to largely determine rates of obesity in western populations; they determine to what extent any inherited tendency to obesity is expressed. As industrialisation produces conditions that increasingly favour excessive weight gain, so more and more people are affected by this problem as more people's threshold of susceptibility is reached – hence the rising prevalence of obesity seen in Europe and the USA. Despite genetic variation in susceptibility to fatness, we are not totally the prisoners of our genes. At the individual level, social class differences in obesity prevalence suggest that many people affect their level of fatness by their behaviour. Our position in society's pecking order of fatness is not so totally pre-ordained by our genes as to make it beyond our own control.

At the population level, if populations re-adopted some of the dietary and lifestyle habits that were the norm just a few years ago, then fatness levels would also fall towards those seen in those earlier years. Likewise, if the obese migrants to the USA and their descendants behaved more like their ancestors in Europe and Asia then fewer of them would be overweight. A relatively low prevalence of obesity is not totally incompatible with living in an affluent, industrial society. The comparatively low levels of obesity and slow rates of increase seen in some affluent countries, such as Sweden, also reinforce this belief. Some groups, such as the Polynesians and Pima Indians, seem to be much more genetically prone to obesity than Caucasians and this would make it particularly difficult for them to maintain low rates of obesity in an affluent, industrialised environment.

In order to reduce obesity, we need to pinpoint which dietary and lifestyle factors trigger it and decide upon their relative importance. Then, we can suggest realistic behaviour changes that will enable people to affect their position within the population pecking order of fatness. We must also identify any policy and environmental factors that encourage people to adopt fattening lifestyles. We must try to reduce the environmental, political or other barriers that prevent people adopting diets and lifestyles that are more conducive to achieving a healthy body weight.

Some specific causes of obesity

In the rest of this chapter, I am going to consider more fully the significance of three factors in the development of obesity, namely:

- ■ 'external' influences upon our food intake;
- ■ diet composition;
- ■ inactivity.

External influences upon food intake

Are obese people more influenced by external factors?

In experimental studies, the food consumption of obese rats and people was more affected than that of lean subjects by several so-called external influences, such as: the ease with which food could be obtained; its palatability; and how anxious the subjects were.

When rats were made to work for their food (by running through a maze) the obese ones ate less than the lean ones, whereas when food was easy to obtain, obese rats ate more than the lean ones. In one ingenious experiment, lean and fat people were offered nuts to eat in a disguised situation. If these nuts were opened and easy to eat, the obese subjects ate many more than the lean ones, but when the subjects had to crack them open for themselves the obese ate far fewer nuts than the lean! In general, if food was easy to obtain and tasted nice then the obese animals and people ate more than the lean. However, when the food was difficult to obtain or did not taste good then the obese ate much less than the lean. The drive to obtain food (hunger) seemed to be reduced in the obese even though they could be persuaded to eat more if the food was tasty and easy to get. Some researchers suggested that the feeding of obese people was more influenced by these external factors than that of lean people whose feeding is accordingly more responsive to their internal physiological mechanisms.

Are obese people less vigilant in monitoring their weight?

It has also been suggested that obese people are less vigilant than lean people in monitoring and regulating their body weight. This might explain the social class differences in obesity rates. It is argued that better educated people from the higher social classes pay more attention to monitoring changes in their body weight and that they take corrective action (eating less and exercising more) before it becomes a major problem. Those from the lower social classes may be less vigilant, so that their condition progresses much further before they become aware of it. Corrective action is now so difficult that it fails. This convinces the person that correction of their condition is beyond their control and so they abandon all attempts at restraint.

One physician has advocated the use of an adjustable waist cord to increase the vigilance of patients. The physician fits the cord so that any increase in waist size beyond the small, patient-adjustable range of the cord, makes it uncomfortable and signals the need for corrective measures. Only the physician can shorten or lengthen the cord beyond this range, for example, when an obese person loses weight. An uncomfortably tight pair of trousers or a tight skirt may serve as a similar early warning signal for many of us!

Do modern diets weaken the link between hunger and eating?

Modern affluent diets are so varied and tempting that we may be persuaded to eat when not hungry and perhaps even to continue eating when our physiological signals should register complete satiation. **Hunger** is the physiological need to eat whilst **appetite** is the hedonistic desire to eat. Appetite may be present despite the absence of hunger and may diminish the role of hunger in the control of feeding.

Increases in the variety of food may encourage overeating. When volunteers rated the pleasantness of different foods, it was found that previous consumption of a food reduced its pleasantness rating, but had little effect on that of other foods – so-called **sensory specific satiety**. When people ate sausages, then, their rating for sausages was reduced but the pleasantness rating for other foods, for example, fruit or cookies was largely unaffected by eating sausages. Subjects offered successive plates of sandwiches ate more if the sandwiches contained different fillings than if they were all the same. More surprisingly, subjects offered successive plates of pasta ate more if the pasta shape was varied than if the shape was the same. Variation in taste or appearance increased the amount eaten. If a diet is monotonous then we are less likely to overeat than if it is varied. This is not too surprising a conclusion – most of us usually 'manage' a little dessert even when satiated by earlier courses of the meal. Even laboratory rats eat much more during cafeteria feeding.

Sensory specific satiety should increase the range of foods that people eat and limit the consumption of any single food. It should therefore decrease the likelihood of nutritional inadequacies because they are unlikely if the diet is varied. It would also reduce the likelihood that any of the toxins found in small amounts in many foods would be consumed in sufficient quantities to be hazardous. In an affluent population, nutrient deficiencies are unlikely, food is always plentiful and its variety appears almost limitless. Under such conditions, sensory specific satiety probably encourages overeating and excessive weight gain.

The effectiveness of food intake control may be compromised because the link between hunger and eating is weakened. We may not wait for our next meal until we are driven by hunger to seek food. We often eat because this is the time in the working day allocated for eating, or because someone has provided a meal for us, or to share a meal we have prepared for our families. If an appetising meal is presented to us before we are overtly hungry then the chances are that we will eat at least some of it. On the other hand, if we are hungry outside normal meal times, then we are quite likely to try and quench this hunger by consuming an energy-rich snack. Hunger is more likely to provoke eating than lack of hunger is to prevent eating.

Analogy with drinking and thirst

Let us consider the simpler link between thirst and drinking. If we only drink plain water and if it requires conscious effort to get water, then thirst is likely to determine how much we drink. But if we have varied and pleasant tasting drinks, some containing drugs like caffeine and alcohol and if many social situations revolve around the consumption of drinks then thirst is no longer the sole determinant of how much we drink. Thirst may compel us to drink but absence of thirst does not stop us from drinking. Even laboratory rats drink much more if their water is sweetened. The man who spends an evening in a bar drinking beer is not merely quenching his thirst. The neighbours who meet each morning for coffee are not motivated primarily by thirst. If we drink too much then we simply excrete the excess but if we eat too much then the surplus calories are stored as fat. We don't just eat because we are hungry; we eat for a variety of social and psychological reasons and so we should not be surprised if our physiological mechanisms for controlling eating are not always effective. Perhaps we should be more surprised that despite this many people stay lean.

Reducing the external triggers to eating

At a practical level, several things should lessen external triggers to eating:

- making food gathering and preparation more arduous;
- decreasing the variety and palatability of food;
- eating only when hungry rather than at times determined by habit or social convention.

Many popular diet books (see Chapter 5) clandestinely use such options by asking readers to 'follow a few simple rules'. These rules often prohibit many of the foods that normally provide most of our calories, making high calorie intake difficult and monotonous. Permitted foods are often expensive, difficult to obtain, require elaborate preparation and of low palatability. Patterns of eating may be prescribed that are inconvenient, not conducive to social eating and make high calorie consumption difficult. If people diligently follow these 'simple rules' then they may well eat less and lose weight even though the rationale offered by the author is nonsense.

Behavioural therapy (see Chapter 6) makes overt use of this approach. Patients are encouraged to identify the external cues that trigger their inappropriate eating and then they take steps to avoid or reduce these external cues. Patients try to make eating a considered, pre-meditated act rather than a subconscious response to circumstances, so snack foods are put on a high shelf or in a locked cupboard so that they have to be actively sought and cannot be subconsciously nibbled.

Diet composition as a cause of obesity

Fats and carbohydrates (sugar and starch) are the major calorie sources and together they supply over 80 per cent of the calories in most diets (the rest comes from protein and alcohol). If a high proportion of calories comes from carbohydrates then a low proportion comes from fat and vice-versa. This is referred to as the **carbohydrate-fat seesaw** – as the proportion of one goes up, so the other goes down. During industrialisation, many carbohydrate calories in the diet are replaced with fat and more of the carbohydrate calories are taken as sugar rather than starch. In some peasant diets, over 75 per cent of the calories come from carbohydrate (mostly starch) with only 10 per cent or less from fat. In the UK and USA, fat accounts for almost 40 per cent of the calories, with carbohydrates down to under 45 per cent. Almost half of these carbohydrate calories may be from sugars. This means that there tends to be not just a carbohydrate-fat seesaw but more specifically a **sugar-fat seesaw** in the diets of Britons and Americans.

In the past, carbohydrates have been blamed for obesity so low carbohydrate diets were recommended for weight loss. Sugar is still seen as something which is particularly liable to encourage weight gain. There is now much evidence to suggest that a high fat diet is more fattening than a high starch or even a high sugar diet. During active weight reduction both fat and sugar need to be reduced. However, the sugar-fat seesaw effect would make a general diet that is low in both fat and sugar difficult to achieve. Fat reduction should be the priority; reduced fat intake has wide health benefits and high fat diets favour weight gain for the reasons listed below.

■ Fat makes diets more energy concentrated; a gram of fat yields nine calories but a gram of sugar or starch only four. Their high energy density is one reason why high fat diets favour weight gain.

■ Fat makes food more palatable. Many of the substances that make food taste and smell good are dissolved in fat. Fat also improves the texture and colour of many foods. Obese people seem to have a greater fat preference than lean people.

■ Calorie for calorie, fat seems to be less satiating than carbohydrate (see Chapter 3). Pre-load meals are meals whose calorie content, timing and composition are controlled by the experimenter and they are used to see the effects of various types of meal on the volunteer's feelings of hunger and satiation and on the amount they eat at their next meal. These studies indicate that fat pre-loads are less satiating and have less effect on the size of the next meal than carbohydrate pre-loads of the same calorie content. The implication is that a snack or meal that is high in carbohydrate is likely to depress your appetite over the following hours by more than one that has an equal number of calories but is high in fat and low in carbohydrate.

■ Excess fat calories can be very efficiently converted to body fat. Only about 4 per cent of the calories in dietary fat are wasted in their conversion to body fat whereas 25 per cent of carbohydrate calories are wasted. In practice, there is little conversion of dietary carbohydrate to body fat on most western diets – dietary carbohydrate is used as an immediate energy source or converted to **glycogen** (animal starch) in the liver and muscles.

Large random surveys indicate that people who obtain the highest proportion of their calories from fat are the most likely to be overweight or obese. Given the carbohydrate-fat and sugar-fat seesaw effects, it follows that people who get more of their calories from carbohydrate and even sugar have a reduced risk of being overweight or obese. In one Scottish survey it was found that the prevalence of overweight and obesity declined as the proportion of calories from carbohydrate or sugar increased, but increased with a growing proportion of calories from fat. Rates of obesity in the 20 per cent of Scots with the highest fat to sugar ratio were much higher than in the 20 per cent with the lowest ratio (3.5 times higher in men and twice as high in women).

In recent years, diets that are high in **dietary fibre** have been widely advocated for improving weight control. Dietary fibre is largely composed of the indigestible forms of carbohydrate and can be found in carbohydrate foods such as starchy cereals and roots, fruits and vegetables. High fibre diets are therefore low in fat, have low energy concentration and are not highly palatable. As high fibre diets are usually low in fat (a fat-fibre seesaw) this would make them less fattening. Fibre also has other effects that aid weight control as listed below.

- ■ Bulky and fibrous foods may make us eat slower.
- ■ Fibre slows stomach emptying, making us feel fuller for longer.
- ■ Fibre slows absorption of food and so prolongs its satiating effects. It also reduces insulin release and prevents the rebound hypoglycaemia (discussed in Chapter 3) that can trigger hunger.

Diets that are low in fat tend to be high in fibre, starch and sugar. People eating such diets tend to be leaner than people eating high fat diets (which are also low in fibre, starch and even sugar). The low energy concentration of low-fat, high-fibre diets is a major reason they help to prevent excessive weight gain. Other factors may make fat more fattening and high fibre foods beneficial for slimmers.

Physical inactivity as a cause of obesity

The need for physical activity continues to decline in the industrialised nations. Car ownership, together with automation in the home, garden and workplace have all combined to minimise the amount of energy that we are required to expend each day. Few people now have physically demanding jobs and increases in leisure time activity (recreational walking, sports and games) have not compensated for this large decrease in required activity. As energy expenditure falls so this also reduces our need for food calories.

Is decreased activity a major reason why obesity rates have risen so sharply in the USA and UK? Do differences in individuals' activity levels make a major contribution to their position in the population pecking order of fatness?

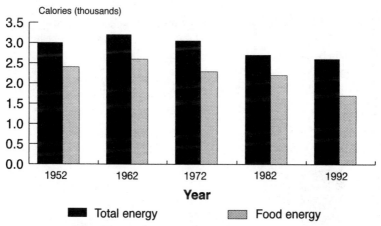

4.1 UK calorie intake

Principal data source: *Diet and cardiovascular disease*. Report on health and social subjects No. 28. London: HMSO 1984

There is evidence that in recent decades Britons and Americans have been eating less but getting fatter. The fall in energy expenditure seems to be outpacing the fall in energy intake. Figure 4.1 shows how estimates of household food consumption and total energy consumption (including alcohol, other drinks, sweets and meals eaten outside the home) changed in Britain over the period 1952–92. Both measures of consumption strongly suggest that the calorie intake of the UK population has been falling for about thirty years. These figures contrast sharply with the rises in average Body Mass Index and steep increases in obesity prevalence over the same period (see Chapter 1). An article published in the *British Medical Journal* in 1995 showed that increases in obesity prevalence in Britain since 1950 have mirrored the increases in car ownership and the number of hours Britons spend watching television. This supports the view that declining activity levels have played a major part in causing the recent large increases in the fatness of Britons and Americans.

Several large British and American surveys have provided support for the proposition that obesity and inactivity tend to go together. In the 1993 *Health Survey for England*, BMI was measured in over sixteen thousand people and activity level was assessed by a questionnaire. Active people were much less likely to be obese than those who were inactive. Physical activity seems to help prevent obesity, and this trend was most pronounced in middle-aged men and women. This is illustrated in Figure 4.2 which shows that in both middle-aged men and women, obesity was more than twice as common amongst those in the lowest activity category as compared to those in the most active categories. Similar US surveys conducted in the early 1970s and early 1980s also indicated that the least active people tended to be the fattest.

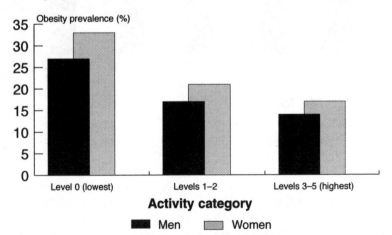

4.2 Obesity prevalence by activity level in middle-aged English people
Data source: *The Health Survey for England 1993*. London: HMSO 1995

In Britain and the USA, obesity is less common in the higher
socioeconomic classes whilst activity levels are higher in these groups.
Table 4.1 shows data from a large nutritional survey conducted in Britain
in the late 1980s. Women in the lower social classes appear to eat less than
higher class women but nonetheless are fatter. At the extremes, these
differences are really quite large. One explanation is that women in the
higher social groups are more active than those in the lower social groups
and so remain leaner despite eating more. Of course, class differences in
the tendency to under record food intake and exaggerate activity is
another possibility.

**Table 4.1   Average BMIs and daily energy intakes in
British women in different social classes**

Data source: *The Dietary and Nutritional Survey of British Adults.*
London: HMSO 1990

	Social class category			
	I & II (high)	III (non-manual)	III (manual)	IV & V (low)
Average BMI	23.8	24.5	24.9	25.8
Energy intake (calories/day)	1740	1710	1670	1580

In surveys conducted in Britain and the USA, it has consistently been
reported that average BMI and obesity prevalence rise with age up until
about the age of 60 (see Chapter 1). There is equally strong evidence that
activity levels decline sharply with age in adults. Is declining activity a
major reason why fatness increases in the middle-aged?

The most popular leisure time pursuit in Britain and America is watching
television, a pursuit that demands physical inactivity. Many people spend
more time watching television than they spend at school or at work.
Rising obesity prevalence in Britain has mirrored the rise in television
viewing hours. One large survey of American children and adolescents
found a strong link between the number of hours of television watched
and the prevalence of obesity. Prevalence of obesity increased with each
extra hour of television watched – a 2 per cent rise in obesity rate per extra
hour of TV watched! Those who watched most TV were also found to be
the most likely to gain weight excessively in the following years.

Simply reducing the amount of television that obese children watch, even without taking any steps to increase activity, is claimed to help them lose weight. If one removes or reduces the inducement to inactivity (television) then there is almost inevitably some increase in activity; they find things to do that use up more energy than passively watching television. It might be even more effective in preventing weight gain in the first place!

Clearly, inactivity and obesity tend to go together. I have suggested that this is because inactivity helps cause obesity but obesity could also cause people to be less active. There is probably an element of truth in both of these possibilities and so one has the makings of a dangerous obesity–inactivity cycle:

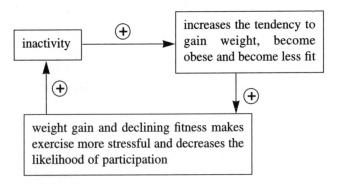

Our activity level has a major effect upon the amount of energy we expend. Inactivity and therefore low energy expenditure must predispose us to excessive weight gain and so an active lifestyle should lessen our chances of becoming obese. Weight reduction programmes that include an exercise element are more likely to produce sustained weight loss than those that do not and regular exercise also has many additional health benefits (see Chapter 6).

Conclusions

■ Evolution has probably left us ill-equipped to cope with an environment where food is plentiful, varied and highly palatable and where there is little requirement for physical activity.

- Both genetic and lifestyle factors contribute to our risk of being obese but recent sharp rises in obesity rates must be due to changes in our diet and/or lifestyle.

- External factors like food palatability, food variety and social/cultural influences upon eating weaken the link between our physiologically controlled hunger drive and our eating behaviour. This makes us prone to overeating and weight gain.

- The composition of our food, particularly its high energy concentration and high fat content, reduces the effectiveness of our physiological control mechanisms and makes us prone to weight gain.

- Rapidly declining activity levels are probably the single most important reason why obesity rates have accelerated so sharply upwards in recent years.

5 | A SURVEY OF DIET BOOKS AND PROGRAMMES

Scope of the chapter

In this chapter, I will critically review a sample of weight loss programmes that have appeared in popular diet books and elsewhere over the last 40 years. I will assess their safety, their likely effectiveness and suggest reasons why many of them may lead to short-term weight loss if followed diligently, even though the reasoning behind them may be flawed. I will offer readers some criteria that they can use to judge weight loss programmes and advisers.

The enormous range of books and strategies

Before starting to write this book, I scoured secondhand shops and markets for diet books. I was surprised at just how plentiful and cheap these discarded diet books were. Many books were in mint condition and multiple copies were usually obtainable. My 'diet library' now contains a fair cross section of the hundreds of diet books published over the last 40 years but cost around the cover price of just one current best seller!

Many of my books claim to have sold millions of copies and most of the authors claim that their method of weight loss is quick, painless and highly successful. Despite this, obesity rates continue to spiral rapidly upwards.

Some authors use their astronomical sales as evidence of the quality of their product – 'so many people would not have bought my book if it did not work!' Professor Tom Sanders of London University has taken a contrasting view and described diet books as a 'capitalist's dream' – a product that does not work but is replaced over and over again by a 'new, improved product'. He goes on to suggest that three features are ideally required for a new and commercially successful diet book:

■ the promise of large and rapid weight loss;

■ a gimmick or magic formula;

■ a slim female author to act as a role model whom the dieter
can aspire to be like.

This book is written by a middle-aged male who struggles to keep his BMI
below the magic 25 figure. It offers no gimmicks and suggests that
sustained weight loss will be a slow and uncomfortable business!

'Celebrity' diets are currently in fashion – any well-known person who
has conspicuously lost weight can increase their wealth still further by
selling us the secret of their success.

Many different strategies for weight loss can be found within my diet
library. The strategies in some books completely contradict those in
others. Food calories come from fats, carbohydrates and proteins and my
books contain contradictory recommendations about the ideal balance of
these three components for dieters. Each of the following has been
recommended by one or more of my books:

■ low carbohydrate;

■ high fat, low carbohydrate;

■ high protein, low carbohydrate and low fat;

■ low fat, high carbohydrate.

Most of the books in my collection offer some scientific or
pseudoscientific rationale for their approach which, despite often being
completely contradictory, may sound equally plausible to non-scientists.
In some cases, these differences in approach represent changes in the
orthodox scientific approach to weight control suggesting that even 'the
experts' have changed their minds.

Do all of these varied diets work?

According to their authors, each of these diverse strategies for weight loss
has been extremely successful. Often the book includes one or more of the
following:

■ case histories of startlingly successful dieters;

■ the results of pseudo-scientific trials of the diet;

■ an account of how the author stumbled upon this amazing
dietary revelation and how this has transformed his/her life.

Is it possible, then, that all or most of these diverse strategies work? The short answer is yes, many of them will probably produce short-term weight loss in people who follow them diligently (although the rates of weight loss claimed by some authors seem improbable). Many of these strategies can produce substantial short-term weight loss, despite the fact that they may be based upon theories and suggested weight loss mechanisms that are incompatible with each other and, in many cases, incompatible with current scientific beliefs. They may succeed in producing weight loss because if they are followed diligently then they are likely to produce a calorie deficit.

Covert ways of reducing energy intake

Most diet books contain sample diet plans and lists of recipes which occupy the bulk of the pages in many books. These diets and recipes are supposed to conform to the rules of the book's diet, although my analysis suggests that in some cases they do not. Many of these diets are designed to be low in calories and this is acknowledged by the author; they represent different ways of supplying the 1000–1500 calories per day that should enable most people to lose weight at a satisfactory rate. These books are often marketed on their 'mouthwatering' low calorie recipes or on their ability to satisfy the appetite despite being low in calories. However, some authors suggest that their diet allows weight loss without the need for calorie restriction – 'provided you stick to a few simple rules then you can lose weight despite eating as much as you want'. These sound particularly attractive to anyone wanting to lose a lot of weight without having to endure the months of discomfort associated with conventional dieting. Some authors suggest that calorie-controlled diets are ineffective and they may even ridicule the idea of calorie restriction as a means of weight control. In practice, however, the book's rules will often produce a calorie deficit for reasons such as those given below.

Forbidding certain foods

The 'few simple rules' in some diet books often involve extensive lists of forbidden or severely restricted foods. Following these 'simple rules' may produce a diet that is actually more restrictive than an orthodox, low-calorie, reducing diet. The prohibited foods in such books usually supply more than half of the calories in current diets and in one extreme case, foods that supply almost 90 per cent of the calories in the average UK and

USA diet are completely prohibited. Figure 5.1 shows a breakdown of the contribution of the main food groups to total calorie intake (this is British data but American results would be fairly similar). These lists of prohibited foods can make it difficult to take in sufficient calories from the permitted foods to maintain energy balance and so people either lose weight or break the diet. If a diet bans foods which normally supply 60 per cent or more of our calories, then it becomes difficult and monotonous to replace these calories by eating more of those foods that are allowed.

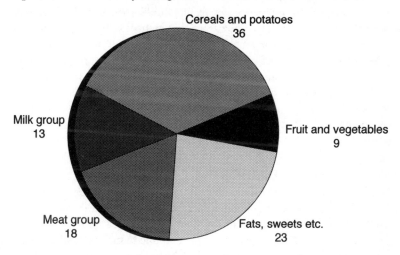

5.1 Contribution of food groups to total calorie intake
Data source: The Dietary and Nutritional Survey of British Adults. London: HMSO 1990.

Giving unlimited access to very low energy foods

Many diets allow almost unlimited quantities of fresh fruit and raw or boiled vegetables to be consumed (excluding starchy vegetables like potatoes). This includes current orthodox reducing diets, i.e. low fat, low sugar, calorie controlled. As we saw in Chapter 4 (p.72) these foods are usually very energy dilute because of their high water content and because they are almost fat-free. Taken together, these foods would normally provide only a few per cent of the calories in British and American diets. A several fold increase in their consumption has a relatively small impact on total calorie intake although the weight of food eaten is much greater. Authors of diet books can therefore justifiably claim that you can eat as much as you want on their plan by allowing unrestricted access to these low energy, bulky foods. Analysis of many of the diet plans in the 'no calorie counting' category of diet books confirms that most of them are, in practice, low in calories.

Making the diet monotonous or of low palatability

Some of the diets recommended in my diet library seem to be of inherently low palatability (at least to my taste). Some authors suggest that you need a period of adjustment for your palate to recover from its assault by modern junk/processed foods before you can appreciate the more subtle flavours and textures in their diet plan. It seems to my cynical eye that the more gushing the author is about their 'delicious' 'mouthwatering' 'satisfying' recipes, the less they appeal to my jaded palate. With other plans, the sheer monotony of the diet would probably discourage high calorie intake after a few days or lead to abandonment of the diet.

If a diet plan removes much of the pleasure of eating, then one should not be too surprised if those people who stick to it eat less as a result. Remember from Chapter 4 that laboratory rats who are given a variety of tasty human foods eat much more than those allowed just the pellet diet? Well some of the diet plans in my books seem to be aiming to almost reverse this process and transfer people onto the human equivalent of the rat's pellet diet! Evidence presented in Chapter 4 also suggested that low palatability may depress calorie intake more in the obese than the lean.

Making eating hard work/expensive

Some diet plans have elaborate rules about the way foods should be prepared and served or recommend substitutes for everyday foods that are difficult to obtain or expensive. It may require much planning, effort and not inconsiderable expense to stick to these rules. Such rules may compound with other factors to reduce total calorie intake.

If eating becomes hard work then this is likely to depress food intake in those people who stick strictly to the rules. It may well be more effective in reducing the food intake of overweight people than it is with lean people. In the last chapter we saw evidence that, in experimental situations, obese rats and people were less inclined to eat if it required effort to get the food. Of course, most people will probably get fed up with the hassle of sticking to the diet and abandon it.

Increasing energy expenditure

Most diet books recommend an increase in physical activity; only the strength and priority attached to this recommendation varies. If this advice is accepted then it will increase energy expenditure and facilitate weight loss. Many recent books contain detailed exercise plans as well as diet plans. Some authors make exaggerated claims about their particular exercise plan just as they do about their diets. Some suggest that their exercises will remove fat from specific regions of the body, some that they have devised exercises that burn fat rapidly without being strenuous; there are even devices that shake or stimulate parts of the body without the need for any active participation by the subject!

If people succeed, even temporarily, in losing weight on their diet, then they usually give at least some credit to their new 'miracle diet'. Most people find it impossible not to break some of the dietary rules and so often accept blame or are blamed for failure. Any successes are used to support the effectiveness of the author's particular gimmick whilst the failures are blamed upon not sticking to the rules.

Whatever the particular gimmick offered by a diet book, then, it is for reasons such as those listed above that people actually lose weight. One could argue that this is partly why orthodox low fat/sugar, high starch/fibre diets work.

- Restricting fat and sugar reduces diet palatability and limits the number of foods that can be eaten freely.
- Limiting access to fatty and sugary foods can increase the effort and/or money required to obtain palatable and culturally normal food; many new 'low fat' and 'low calorie' convenience foods are relatively expensive.
- Energy dilute foods can be eaten freely and should replace some energy concentrated foods.
- Encouraging activity is part of good orthodox regimes.

If an unorthodox diet may work then why shouldn't I use it?

Many unorthodox diets may achieve weight loss but they are considered undesirable for a number of reasons.

The diet is not sustainable

Some diets are unpalatable, monotonous, very different from the normal cultural eating pattern or just plain bizarre. Determined individuals may be able to follow them for a while but, in the longer term, they are incompatible with a normal, healthy and economically realistic family diet. They may achieve considerable weight loss if followed strictly by highly committed individuals who are prepared to put up with the inconvenience and discomfort, but the same could be said of any low calorie diet sheet given by a doctor or dietitian. The difficulties and discomfort associated with calorie restriction may be masked by the difficulties and discomfort of sticking to the particular rules and philosophy of the plan. Some people actually like a set of clear and rigid rules, because they know exactly what is expected of them and are not given any options or difficult decisions to make. However, in the longer term, only those who become 'converts' and follow the dietary regime with an evangelical fervour will sustain any initial weight losses. These converts may actually thrive upon the strict rules and restrictions which may give them a purpose in life and enhance their feelings of individuality. However, most purchasers of the book will not become converts – they are prepared to try the plan, often rather half-heartedly, because they are hoping for some magic formula that will make them lose weight without much effort or commitment on their part. Such people will not lose weight whatever strategy is used and so their book will be discarded and replaced by the latest entry into the diet best seller charts.

Short-term hazards

When eating normally, the brain uses carbohydrate (glucose) as its source of energy. After a few hours of fasting, however, carbohydrate stores are used up and the brain cannot switch over to using fat as many other tissues do. Some glucose can be made from protein but this process is inefficient and depletes muscles and essential organs. Therefore, during prolonged fasting the liver produces substances called **ketones** from fat and these can be used by the brain as an alternative to glucose. During severe energy or carbohydrate restriction, these ketones accumulate in the blood and give the breath an alcohol-like smell. This **ketosis** upsets the normal acid-base balance of the blood and leads to increased loss of minerals in urine. It also produces light-headedness and altered psychological functioning which could, possibly, help to trigger eating disorders.

Ketosis is a natural response to starvation, but starvation is an 'adverse circumstance' and so one should not assume that ketosis is a totally benign condition. A very severe ketosis occurs in uncontrolled, insulin-dependent diabetes and is largely responsible for the potentially fatal diabetic coma. Some advocates of ketosis-inducing diets argue that ketosis is actually an advantage of their diet. They argue that it reduces hunger, that some people find the light-headedness quite a pleasant sensation and that the production of ketones is a tangible indicator of fat breakdown. However, low carbohydrate diets that are associated with ketosis and other metabolic disturbances are not recommended by nutritionists today. Diets that are too low in calories also lead to rapid loss of lean tissue and this is also undesirable. The rapid weight loss they achieve is deceptive because much of the extra weight lost, as compared to more moderate diets, is lean tissue and water rather than fat.

Long-term hazards

Some popular diet books have advocated diets that are undesirable or even unsafe on wider health grounds. Most obviously, some are inadequate in vitamins or minerals and so require the use of supplements to prevent deficiency. As we eat less on a diet then this predisposes us to deficiencies and this risk is amplified if the range of foods is restricted. Any diet that forbids a whole food group, as listed below, is thus considered nutritionally unsound:

- the milk group (milk, milk products, yoghurt, cheese and vegetarian milks);
- the meat group (meat, fish, eggs) *and vegetarian alternatives (such as peas, beans and nuts)*;
- the cereal group (rice, bread, pasta, breakfast cereals and foods made from grains);
- the fruit and vegetable groups.

Good orthodox reducing diets often increase the intake of essential nutrients because they replace some high energy/low nutrient foods with some that are low energy/high nutrient. Supplements will prevent deficiency of known vitamins/minerals but may not contain other substances in foods that may have beneficial effects upon our long-term health.

Other diets may be at variance with a healthy long-term dietary pattern. British and American adults are currently being advised that they should eat less fat, less sugar, more starch and more fibre than they currently do. To achieve this they will need to:

- eat more cereals, fruits and vegetables;
- moderate their use of foods from the meat and milk groups (particularly limiting the fattier products in these categories like whole milk and fatty meat);
- make only sparing use of fats, oils, sugar and foods/drinks that are high in fat or sugar.

Clearly diets that severely restrict carbohydrate intake (and therefore cereals and potatoes) are incompatible with this advice, as are diets that specifically advocate increases in fat consumption. High fat intake is now believed to be linked to increased risk of heart disease, strokes, some cancers, diabetes as well as increased risk of weight gain. Low carbohydrate diets are almost inevitably high fat diets (the carbohydrate-fat seesaw).

Diets that are very high in protein are also considered undesirable; in the long-term, there is speculation about whether they may increase the risk of kidney failure. Britons and Americans are specifically recommended, on general health grounds, not to consume diets that are very high in protein. The safe upper limits recommended for protein intake are not too far above current intakes and so large increases are undesirable.

Case studies of particular diet books

In this section I give some examples of books that illustrate many of the weight loss strategies that have been popular over the last 40 years.

Low carbohydrate diets

There are many variations on the 'low carbohydrate' theme in my diet library. The high fat and high protein diets (discussed next) are variations on the low carbohydrate theme. My example of a low carbohydrate diet is from a book written by an eminent British professor of nutrition in the 1950s. It remained in print for several decades and was very influential. The idea that carbohydrates, and starchy foods in particular, should be severely restricted during dieting still persists to this day even though it is contrary to the current scientific consensus.

Readers of the book are advised to severely restrict the intake of carbohydrate (both starches and sugars). The author suggests that as carbohydrate provides over half of the dietary energy directly (in the 1950s) and is also needed to carry much of the dietary fat (e.g. butter/margarine spread on bread, fat carried by fried foods, fat in cakes and pies etc.) then this carbohydrate restriction will also, in practice, reduce absolute fat consumption and consequently reduce total calorie intake. Although the proportion of calories derived from fat is expected to rise on this diet (because of the carbohydrate-fat seesaw), the actual number of grams/ounces of fat eaten may actually fall.

Readers are advised to start with a diet containing only 75 g of carbohydrate which is about a third as much as is currently consumed by a typical Briton or American eating 2000 calories per day and only about a quarter of what such a person would be recommended to consume. Foods such as meat, fish, eggs, green vegetables, cheese, butter, cream, oils and other fats are almost carbohydrate-free and are not restricted. High carbohydrate foods like bread, rice, pasta, sugar and milk are severely restricted and even fruits are restricted because most contain some natural sugar. This diet almost stands current nutritional guidelines on their head.

The diet did seem to achieve considerable short-term successes with people who followed it. At the time the book was first written, the current belief that high fat and saturated fat intake are implicated in the development of heart disease was not well established. In my 1965 edition, the author does acknowledge this concern but suggests that overweight and inactivity are more important causes of heart disease than is the fat content of the diet. Even today, many nutritionists would sympathise with this assessment.

This author acknowledges that weight loss only occurs if calorie intake is reduced or expenditure increased through exercise. He uses carbohydrate restriction as a means of reducing total calorie intake because severe carbohydrate restriction makes it difficult to consume excess calories. He also believed that fat was more satiating than carbohydrate because it delayed stomach emptying, something that was generally accepted at the time. This author does not actively promote increased fat intake and expects that the absolute amount of fat eaten will either stay the same or go down.

Specifically high fat diets

One book in my collection specifically recommends increased fat intake. The author claims that high fat intake will stimulate metabolism and 'burn off' surplus calories. He claims that men eating up to 2600 calories per day can still lose weight if their carbohydrate intake is low enough (many reducing diets aim for 1000–1500 calories per day). People should thus be able to lose weight with little or no restriction upon their calorie intake provided they are eating a high fat, low carbohydrate diet.

As in the previous book there are lists of low carbohydrate foods that can be eaten freely when dieting. They include beef dripping, butter, cream cheese, cream and most fatty meats provided that both the fat and lean are eaten. Most green vegetables, salad vegetables and other low carbohydrate vegetables can also be eaten freely. Only a few fruits can be eaten freely on this diet, most are restricted because of their sugar content. The forbidden and severely restricted foods normally contribute around 60 per cent of the calories in the normal UK diet, including, for example:

- bread and cereals (including cakes, biscuits, rice, pasta and breakfast cereals);
- potatoes, and other high carbohydrate vegetables;
- many meat and fish products that contain cereals, such as sausages, pies and those that are breaded or battered;
- foods/drinks with added sugar;
- most alcoholic drinks except dry wine;
- milk (especially low fat milk!) and many milk products.

Even this 60 per cent figure does not include the fat that is largely dependent upon consumption of the banned/restricted foods, for example, the fat spread on bread, the fat eaten with fried potatoes.

The central thesis of this book is that there is a large capacity to burn off surplus calories i.e. **adaptive thermogenesis**. According to this author, in people prone to weight gain, this burning off process is activated by fat but not by carbohydrate; surplus fat calories are burnt off whereas surplus carbohydrate calories are stored as fat. He believed that only carbohydrates fatten people. Current evidence indicates that fat intake has much less effect on metabolism than carbohydrate intake and that fat is actually more fattening than carbohydrate.

The author promotes a high fat diet but if one actually follows his rules, that is, a very low carbohydrate intake (60 g target) and a ratio of three grams of protein to each gram of fat, then the resulting diet would actually be very low in carbohydrate and high in protein but the proportion of calories derived from fat would not be dissimilar from current average diets. The author's own sample diet plans do not follow the three grams of protein to one of fat rule. By my analysis, the sample diets are very low in carbohydrate and fibre as intended by the author and fat actually makes up a very high proportion of the calories (around 55 per cent). By my estimations, these sample diets are also quite low in calories, average intake would be well under 2000 calories per day, with some days as low as 1500 calories. Despite the apparently liberal use of high calorie fatty foods, the calorie intake is low enough for an average man burning over 2500 calories per day to lose weight steadily. As predicted in the previous example, the absolute amount of fat may be slightly less than is currently consumed by an average British man. The sample diets contain adequate amounts of the major vitamins and minerals.

High protein diets

The diets in both of the previous categories would result in relatively high protein intakes. However, one book in my diet library specifically aims to maximise the protein content of the diet. The recommended diet is virtually carbohydrate-free and also eliminates all visible fat and added fat from the diet. The only permitted foods on this diet are lean meats, skinned chicken and turkey, white fish (not oily fish), shellfish, eggs, cottage cheese or other cheese made from skimmed milk. No other foods are permitted and even minor lapses such as the sugar in a piece of gum are considered significant! These permitted foods probably contribute not much more than 10 per cent of the calories to the usual diet. The following day's intake would seem to be consistent with the rules and spirit of the plan:

Breakfast   large portion smoked haddock (150 g)
2 boiled eggs

Snack   pot of low fat cottage cheese (45 g)

Lunch   large steak (210 g – lean only)
2 eggs (poached or fried without fat)
smear of tomato ketchup

Snack   pot of cottage cheese

Dinner   prawns (40 g) with small amount (15 g) of cocktail sauce
                 (ketchup and low calorie mayonnaise)
                 large portion (200 g) of skinned roast chicken

Beverages   at least 4 pints of water; unlimited amounts of tea/coffee
                 without milk or sugar and diet soft drinks (artificial
                 sweeteners are allowed).

This represents well under 1500 calories and over 60 per cent of those
calories come from protein, as compared with 15 per cent of calories from
protein in typical USA and UK diets. The diet is almost carbohydrate-free
and fat contributes about 37 per cent of the calories which is similar to
typical diets but it is much richer in saturated fat and cholesterol than current
diets. This diet has almost no dietary fibre, carotene or vitamin C and is very
low in calcium, vitamin B1 and vitamin A. Such deficiencies are inevitable
with such a narrow range of permitted foods. People are encouraged to use
this diet for weeks or even months until they reach their target weight. A
daily vitamin and nutrient supplement is recommended but even so most
nutritionists would regard this diet as very unsound and undesirable.

'Avoid a few foods' diets

One of my books suggests that in order to lose weight, all one needs to do
is to eliminate four foods from the diet. This sounds too good to be true
and, of course, it is – the four foods to be avoided are wheat, milk, sugar
and potatoes and anything that contains these ingredients. Other plants of
the potato family are also banned, for example, tomatoes, peppers and
aubergines. It is also recommended that margarine and oils should be kept
to a minimum with the exception of costly extra virgin olive oil. Foods
that contain these ingredients probably account for over 70 per cent of the
calories in the average diet. Even then, the author concedes that if people
eat enough of the permitted high calorie foods then they may still not lose
weight. She recommends extra measures in such circumstances, for
example, adding all other grains to the list of forbidden foods, use of a
specifically low calorie version of the basic plan, including some 'fast
days' or taking more exercise. The simple avoidance of four foods has
resulted in a regime that is far more restrictive and difficult to implement
than any conventional diet.

Gimmicks and bizarre diets

Over the years, numerous new gimmick diets have become immensely popular for a few months, made their authors a fortune and then rapidly disappeared into obscurity. Often these diets focus on some particular food or foods, such as grapefruit, and these foods are attributed with almost magical properties such as the ability to stimulate the breakdown of body fat or to accelerate metabolism.

Some books offer diet plans that are so far removed from the normal eating pattern that they can only be classified as bizarre. A cynic might suggest that the more bizarre and improbable the diet is, then the more likely it is to be popularised by the media and to make the author's fortune.

One book includes dozens of what the authors themselves call 'bizarre one-dimensional diets' in which subjects are restricted to eating just one food or very few foods. These diets are inevitably deficient in essential nutrients, monotonous and contrary to the most fundamental principle of sound nutrition – diversity. A vitamin-mineral supplement is recommended and it is suggested that they are unsuitable for those with a 'medical condition'. Nevertheless, healthy people are encouraged to believe that it is acceptable to keep to these bizarre diets for anything up to two months! For example:

- the buttermilk only diet – just six glasses of buttermilk daily;
- the cottage cheese and grapefruit diet – six moderate portions of grapefruit and cottage cheese each day;
- the eggs and tomatoes diet – up to six hard boiled eggs and six small tomatoes each day!

Why are intelligent people prepared to even consider such manifestly bizarre and unnatural diets? One reason is that they leave absolutely no margin for error; there is no doubt about what is or is not consistent with the rules and if one can bear to stick to the rules then one will lose weight. This is also the major attraction of many meal replacement diet products – 'a special, scientifically formulated and delicious' cookie, candy bar, milk shake or soup is consumed instead of a normal meal. The calorie counting and decision making is done by the manufacturer rather than the consumer. Marketing of these products usually emphasises their added nutrients and their low calorie content compared to normal meals. However, these products are usually expensive and may contain just as many calories as an ordinary cookie or candy bar.

Food combining diets

Several books use the '**food combining**' principle devised by an American physician, Dr William Hay, early in this century. Hay attributed disease to overproduction and accumulation of toxins, especially the 'acid products of digestion and metabolism' leading to acid poisoning of the body. He argued that health could be improved by adopting a diet and lifestyle that (a) reduced production and increased elimination of these 'acid toxins' and (b) involved consumption of more alkali-producing foods. In order to achieve these ends one needs to:

- reduce consumption of acid-producing foods (proteins, starches and refined foods);
- increase intake of fruits, vegetables and salads;
- not eat fruits at main meals;
- not mix together foods that are high in protein (e.g. meat, fish, eggs and milk) with foods that are high in carbohydrate (e.g. cereals and potatoes).

It is this last point, the need to separate foods of different types, that is the highly controversial and defining feature of food combining diets. This separation of protein and carbohydrates is said to be necessary because carbohydrates require an alkaline medium for their digestion in the gut whereas proteins require an acid medium for their digestion. Modern versions of the 'Hay' diet define high protein and high carbohydrate as 'more than 20 per cent' which gets around the problem that many natural foods contain both protein and carbohydrate but few would contain more than 20 per cent of each.

Most nutritionists would classify food combining as a fad diet and believe that its central tenet is false. Our gut is perfectly capable of digesting carbohydrate and protein mixtures; the acid-alkali balance of the gut contents change as they pass through the gut. Strictly following one of the diet plans in the most recent of my food combining diet books (1993) would probably lead to some weight loss because it would, in practice, reduce calorie intake for several of the 'hidden' reasons listed earlier. For adults, I see no major nutritional objections to the diet – it uses all of the major food groups (although at separate meals), it includes adequate amounts of essential nutrients, carbohydrate and fibre and is not high in saturated fat. I would not recommend using this diet as the basis for feeding rapidly growing children.

As a consumer, and someone who enjoys social eating, I would not for one moment contemplate adopting this diet in preference to a conventional reducing diet. Advocates of food combining concede that it is a completely different way of eating. Most people would find it difficult, inconvenient and probably expensive to implement this new way of eating. It would greatly reduce the pleasure of eating – it's a diet for 'converts'. Despite claims to the contrary, there is a large number of foods to avoid in my latest version of a food combining diet for weight reduction, and these foods account for a high proportion of usual calorie intake, for example:

- almost all processed foods;
- beef and pork and all products made from them;
- anything containing white flour or cornflour;
- all sweets, candies, chocolate, preserves;
- beer and spirits.

Even more restrictive is the fact that most of the 'culturally normal' European and American meals are banned by the rules, for example:

- breakfast cereals with milk;
- cheese, meat, egg or fish sandwiches;
- pasta with meat, fish or cheese sauce;
- potatoes or rice with meat, fish, eggs or cheese;
- hamburger in a bun;
- pizza.

To devise a satisfying and acceptable diet excluding these foods and these combinations requires pretty single-minded commitment.

No food diets

These are the so-called **very low calorie diets** (VLCDs). Commercial products that are 'scientifically formulated' to contain all of the essential vitamins and minerals but provide only 400-800 calories per day. The product is consumed as a flavoured drink and is used to replace normal food. It is very difficult, using normal food, to provide all of the essential nutrients in so few calories. Sometimes a cheaper 'milk diet' is used as an alternative to these commercial products, for example, skimmed or semi-skimmed milk plus a multivitamin and mineral supplement. These VLCDs are an extension of the meal replacement cookies, candy bars and shakes that were mentioned earlier. Apart from fasting, this is the most extreme dietary intervention for weight loss. The attraction for dieters is that they are absolved of all responsibility for food choice – the regime is very clearly prescribed, significant mistakes are not possible and weight loss must occur if one sticks to the regime. For people who comply with these regimes then they do produce substantial and fairly rapid weight loss. The disadvantages of these regimes are also pretty clear and some are listed below.

- ■ The user gets no experience of eating a real diet that is capable of maintaining any short-term weight losses induced by this 'controlled starvation', and they are likely to regain any weight as soon as control of their eating is returned to them. It has been argued that this could be viewed as an advantage of these products because it minimises contact with food and breaks bad eating habits.
- ■ The rapid weight loss leads to high loss of lean tissue. It is difficult to measure this change in body composition accurately and some advocates of these products claim that this problem has been exaggerated.
- ■ The energy deficit is so severe that **ketosis** occurs.
- ■ This 'controlled starvation' risk might precipitate an eating disorder.
- ■ It is potentially dangerous, especially if used for prolonged periods without proper supervision.

Most nutritionists would not recommend these products for unsupervised use by the average dieter. They are an extreme measure that is inappropriate for people who are only moderately overweight. The commercial motivation may persuade some unscrupulous 'counsellors' to recommend them to people who are not even overweight. Some nutritionists do consider that these products may have a role in the supervised treatment of people with moderate or severe obesity (BMI well in excess of 30) which poses a larger threat to health.

High starch, low fat diets

This approach, coupled with increased exercise, is the orthodox approach to weight control. Indeed, diets of this general type are now recommended for all adults and schoolchildren, irrespective of whether or not they need to lose weight. A few of the newer books in my diet library recommend this approach without any frills, although many try to be distinctive by the use of a gimmick or a celebrity author. Many of these books are filled up with:

- ■ 'personal discovery' stories, case histories and trials of the diet;
- ■ practical advice on how to lower fat/sugar intakes and increase the prominence of starch/fibre in the diet, including the author's own 'unique recipe collection and meal plans';
- ■ practical advice about how to increase activity often including the author's own 'unique exercises or workout plan'.

I also advocate this approach and as I am going to give my own tips for increasing activity and reducing fat/calorie intake in Chapter 6, I will therefore say no more about this strategy here.

High fibre diets

Increasing dietary fibre is a dominant theme in several diet books. One author attributes almost magical weight control properties to fibre. Diets that are naturally high in fibre would be recommended by most nutritionists for reasons such as those listed below:

- ■ they are inevitably low in fat and high in starch (the fibre-fat seesaw);
- ■ they are bulky (low energy density) partly because they are low in fat;
- ■ fibre may prolong the satiating power of food by slowing its absorption to produce a 'slow-release' effect;
- ■ diets naturally high in fibre tend to be nutrient rich;
- ■ fibre improves bowel function.

High fibre intakes and sudden increases in fibre consumption may cause flatulence, bloating and diarrhoea and make life very uncomfortable at least for a while. Very high intakes of fibre may reduce vitamin and mineral absorption although this will not be a problem if the fibre is a natural part of the foods that are eaten. Adding concentrated fibre to foods amplifies the problems and minimises the benefits. Bran and concentrated fibres are unpalatable and so bran-enriched foods often contain large amounts of sugar and/or salt to make them edible. Eating more naturally fibre-rich foods lowers the fat content and energy density of the diet, but adding bran to a high fat dish does not lower its fat content, nor make it less fattening or healthier. Naturally high-fibre diets are generally a good diet choice which I would recommend, but adding liberal amounts of bran to your current diet or liberal use of fibre-enhanced foods will be ineffective and may simply lead to flatulence, bloating and diarrhoea.

Assessing your new diet book or programme

How do you decide whether the plan recommended in your new book or by your new diet counsellor is likely to be safe, effective and sustainable? How do you decide which new diet book amongst the dozens in your local bookshop (or secondhand shop!) you should try?

Negative indicators

Watch out for the following:

- The diet is monotonous and/or unappetising. Remember you may need to follow the plan for many weeks or months.
- The diet requires a 'whole new approach' to eating and is incompatible with social eating except with other converts. Are you prepared for conversion?
- Whole food groups are banned. This diet is nutritionally unsound; even if a diet is intended for vegetarians it should use the vegetarian alternatives in the meat and milk groups.
- Dietary supplements are recommended. This is an admission that the diet is nutritionally inadequate. If specific brands of supplements are advocated or expensive supplements are supplied by your counsellor then this is probably commercially motivated.
- Passive exercisers, slimming belts, or other aids are suggested. Likewise if there is promotion of some new wonder product that will: prevent absorption or digestion of food; mobilise fat or stimulate metabolism; have some other unspecified weight reducing effect. Treat any claims for such products with extreme caution. Is the book or

counselling programme primarily a medium for selling ineffective and expensive junk products?

- Beware of diets that specifically reduce intakes of starchy foods or fruits and vegetables.
- Beware of diets that specifically aim to increase protein intakes, for example, by using very large amounts of meat, eggs, fish, skimmed milk.
- The diet recommends expensive or unusual ingredients that are difficult to obtain. Extra virgin olive oil gets a very good press in my diet library and, although I am an olive oil fan, it has just as many calories as other oils but at ten times the price.
- Beware of exaggerated claims about anticipated rates of weight loss and that substantial weight loss can be achieved without any hardship, for example, 'Magic diet, lose up to 30 pounds in 30 days – no hunger'.
- Beware of claims that a particular programme can 'spot reduce' fat from particular regions of the body.
- Beware of programmes that use unqualified advisers as 'counsellors' and of diet book authors whose only expertise is in journalism, self publicity or making money. In the UK, **State Registered Dietitian (SRD)** is a formal dietetics qualification **(Registered Dietitian (RD)** in the USA). In America, dietitions with a licence to practise may use the initials LD (Licensed Dietitian). The terms nutritionist, nutrition counsellor and dietist may be used by people without any formal qualifications. A nutritionist is simply someone who has studied nutrition or claims to have studied it! Readers are advised to check whether their adviser has any recognised qualification from a recognised academic institution, for example, Bachelor of Science (BS or BSc), Master of Science (MS or MSc); a science doctorate (Doctor of Philosophy or PhD), a medical qualification (MD or MB, ChB) or a nursing qualification (RN or RGN). These formal qualifications are not a guarantee of appropriate knowledge but they are a positive sign.

Be aware

Regard with extreme scepticism:

- The first few chapters of the book which deal with the author's personal discovery story, case histories of amazingly successful dieters and/or pseudo-scientific trials of the plan.
- Any claims to have developed 'a new and exciting range of mouthwatering recipes that make dieting a pleasure'. Look at some of these recipes and try to imagine the taste and texture of the end-product!

Positive indicators

The following points would suggest a sensible diet:

- The diet uses foods from all the major food groups and is generally varied.
- The diet is a recognisable variation of a 'normal' diet. It includes foods that you could offer to non-dieting friends and be confident of them visiting again. It is a diet that can be adjusted at the point of delivery (the table) to meet the differing needs of the whole household including lean and active growing children.
- It is acknowledged that calorie deficit is required for weight loss.
- Fat consumption is preferentially reduced (also sugar and alcohol).
- Fruits and vegetables are used liberally.
- Starchy foods are only limited because overall calorie intake is controlled – they are more prominent as a proportion of the diet than they are in your current diet.
- The predicted rates of weight loss are much less than you had hoped for.
- There is proper emphasis given to increased activity as an adjunct to dieting; extra marks if there is a section detailing practical hints on how to increase your activity.

Conclusions

- Many diverse strategies have been suggested for losing weight. The advice in some books is the complete opposite of that in others.
- Many of these strategies may produce initial weight loss despite being based upon false theory because, in practice, the advice will lead to reduced calorie intake.
- Many of these weight loss strategies produce diets that are inadequate in essential nutrients, or are likely to have adverse consequences upon health in the short- or long-term.
- Readers should use the criteria offered in this chapter to decide whether any weight loss programme is likely to be safe and effective and whether their diet counsellor/adviser is really qualified to provide dietary advice.

6 HOW CAN I LOSE WEIGHT?

Scope of the chapter

In this chapter, I have tried to outline some broad principles for achieving and sustaining weight loss with the aim of empowering readers to devise their own 'lifestyle' plan for weight control. Devising a diet and exercise programme is not difficult but keeping to it is. Many existing plans conform to the principles laid out in this chapter but are often unsuccessful because people do not stick to them. To have the best chance of success, a weight loss programme should ideally take account of factors such as:

- your likes, dislikes and food intolerances;
- your beliefs and cultural values;
- your pattern of eating;
- your economic circumstances;
- your food preparation skills and facilities;
- your need to fit your diet in with the needs of others;
- your amount of leisure time, your access to leisure time facilities and your personal activity preferences;
- your ability and willingness to incorporate more exercise into the activities of everyday living.

A weight loss programme that takes account of these factors and is tailored to your circumstances should have the best chance of success. You may therefore be the best person to design your weight loss plan.

However, for those who feel the need to seek out professional help with their weight loss then their family physician is probably the most obvious starting place for that search. S/he may provide help directly or should be able to direct you towards other practitioners specialising in particular forms of treatment. The telephone directory should contain lists of local slimming clubs, therapists and self-help groups.

I have identified increasing activity as an important element in weight control, especially in the prevention of weight gain and its regain after dieting. I have advocated a diet that is low in fat but relatively rich in starchy foods and in fruits and vegetables. Such a diet is conducive to weight loss, but in its general nature is suitable for non-dieting adults and older children. I have suggested a number of changes that can contribute to increasing activity and to reducing fat and calorie intake.

Should I be trying to lose weight?

The general dietary pattern suggested in this chapter is appropriate and desirable for most healthy adults and older children and very few of us would not benefit from being more active. A reduced fat diet, when coupled with an active lifestyle, should be conducive to weight maintenance or even gradual loss without the continual need for severe food deprivation and calorie counting. However, deliberate calorie restriction to produce energy deficit may be undesirable for some people and so before embarking upon any weight loss programme you should look back to Chapter 2 (p.44) and consider whether this is appropriate for you; if you are in any doubt then seek professional guidance.

I would especially remind parents of my earlier advice to seek professional guidance before putting growing children onto a calorie-restricted diet. A moderately low fat, low sugar diet is appropriate and desirable for school-aged children but I would see the increasing levels of childhood obesity as primarily a problem caused by inactivity rather than diet composition.

Our natural control mechanisms should ensure that healthy adults eat enough calories to maintain adequate energy reserves, and this general diet and lifestyle can be safely used by most adults, even if they do not need to lose weight, provided they do not resist their hunger drive and consciously restrict their food intake.

There is no magic formula

There are no effortless or painless ways of losing substantial amounts of weight. All of the current slimming pills, devices and surgical procedures for weight loss are of limited effectiveness. Many carry significant risks and should only be contemplated in extreme cases. Many weight loss products and devices are frankly fraudulent.

Substantial weight loss requires the body to be in prolonged energy deficit but we have evolved very efficient mechanisms that drive us to eat enough food to prevent energy deficit. Our control mechanisms may permit, or even encourage, overeating but nature makes energy deficit very uncomfortable. When we diet we are trying to resist these powerful, natural drives that normally prevent energy deficit. Appetite suppressant drugs may reduce these drives, psychotherapy may help us to resist them and dietary manipulations may maximise the satiating power of each food calorie. Ultimately, however, the dieter is still going to have to endure considerable discomfort and exercise considerable willpower to lose a lot of weight. Despite this pessimistic conclusion and despite all of the difficulties, anyone who does achieve prolonged energy deficit will lose weight. Weight loss is not impossible for anyone if they are determined enough, persistent enough and if they have a sound weight loss programme.

Success or failure?

The responsibility for the success or failure of any weight loss programme ultimately lies with the dieter rather than the therapist or advisor. The 'professional' can only empower and encourage the dieter. This is a difficult concept for many 'patients' and professionals to accept. Normally, when we consult a doctor about an injury or illness, our role as patient is seen as a largely passive one – we are required merely to take the prescribed drugs or submit to the prescribed surgery. Any control over outcome is seen to be largely in the hands of the expert. Even though the patient may be required to make some contribution to treatment by sticking to the treatment plan or making some lifestyle changes, the professional's skill in selecting and carrying out the correct treatment is seen as the crucial factor for a successful recovery.

Overweight and obesity are at the opposite end of this spectrum of control. In this case, the expert can usually do no more than provide information, advice and encouragement. The success or failure of the treatment depends largely upon the patient's ability to understand, interpret and successfully implement the treatment plan. Acceptance of this fact is crucial to success. Even when obese patients are confined to metabolic wards, where food and drink intake are directly controlled by medical staff, patients have prevented successful treatment by consuming extra food smuggled into the hospital. Some patients who have had their stomach size reduced by 90 per cent by surgical stapling still manage to consume enough to prevent successful weight loss!

There are many barriers to successful implementation of a weight reduction plan:

- the treatment rules are often complicated – deciding on what and how much you are permitted to eat is not always easy;
- any benefits may take a long time to emerge because substantial loss of weight may take weeks;
- the 'costs' of treatment are high – dieting is uncomfortable and inconvenient.

Anyone attempting to lose a lot of weight must be prepared to accept that the responsibility for success or failure is largely theirs and that they will have to endure prolonged discomfort to achieve success. If you expect the latest best selling diet book to offer you an easy and painless way to lose weight – 'lose weight without really trying', 'the pounds will just drop off' – then you are destined for disappointment and your new miracle diet book will probably join countless others at the local fleamarket. Half-hearted attempts at dieting are pointless, they will incur much of the discomfort of a successful programme but will merely bring disappointment and lower self-esteem when they fail. We all know someone who is on a semi-permanent, half-hearted diet but never seems to lose any weight. Enthusiasm and effort should be concentrated into fewer but hopefully more successful efforts.

Losing a lot of weight takes time

Many popular diet books suggest rates of weight loss that seem to be impossible – 'lose up to 30 pounds in 30 days.'

It may have taken many years to accumulate large amounts of excess fat, so one should not expect to be able to get rid of it in a few days. The object of dieting is to lose fat but to minimise loss of lean tissue. Some loss of lean tissue should and will occur during weight loss because obese people have more lean tissue as well as more fat and even fat tissue has some 'lean' in it. A rule of thumb is that weight loss in obese people should be roughly 25 per cent lean and 75 per cent fat to maintain a normal body composition. During gradual weight loss in obese people this ideal is roughly achieved but those tempted by crash diets should be aware that more severe dieting increases the proportion of lean that is lost. A combination of diet and exercise seems to protect lean tissue and a higher proportion of any losses are fat.

Beware extreme diets

In a classic experiment, young men were put onto a very severe diet (600 calories per day) and were required to maintain their activity in order to achieve an estimated daily energy deficit of about 2000 calories. These men lost about five pounds (1 kg is equivalent to about two pounds) each over the first three days of this regime but less than one-and-a-half pounds of this was fat. The total weight loss after a fortnight on this regime was 14 pounds but only about five-and-a-half pounds of this weight loss was fat, the rest was lean tissue including over six pounds of water. Rate of weight loss declined sharply as the diet proceeded but fat loss remained fairly constant – the 'quality' of the weight loss increased with time. Even this extreme and unsustainable regime achieved a rate of fat loss of less than three pounds per week. Men on a less severe regime which allowed them just over 1000 calories per day lost almost as much fat as the more restricted men but much less lean. On the severe regime much of the extra weight lost compared to the more moderate regime was lean tissue and its associated water.

Two pounds (1 kg) of fat tissue yields somewhere around 7000 calories. To lose this fat in a week, one therefore needs to have a daily energy deficit of 1000 calories. To achieve this, a small and inactive young woman would probably have to consume much less than 1000 calories per day. During the first few days of a starvation diet, the body's small store of glycogen (animal starch) is depleted. The total stores of glycogen are only about a pound (0.5 kg) but loss of this glycogen also results in the loss of over three pounds (1.5 kg) of associated water. This means that an energy deficit of only 500 calories is necessary to produce a pound (0.5 kg) of weight loss by this route. However, as soon as the diet is moderated, the glycogen stores will be replenished and this weight regained; only around 500 surplus calories are required to regain a pound (0.5 kg) by this route. Lean tissue also contains about 75 per cent water and so loss of a pound of lean tissue, such as muscle, also requires an energy deficit of only about 500 calories. Very rapid weight loss suggests that lean tissue and water is being lost. These figures also have their bright side; it takes much more than 7000 calories to put on two pounds of fat and this means that the *occasional* lapse in a diet will not undo weeks of hard work and lead to instant, large fat regain (see **catastrophising** later in the chapter).

How long to reach your target weight?

It is reasonable to aim for an energy deficit of somewhere between 500 and 1000 calories per day. If this is achieved then the rate of weight loss after the first week or two should be around one to two pounds (0.5–1kg) each week. Whether you should aim for the top or bottom of this range will depend upon your energy needs. If they are low (for example, a small, inactive woman) you should aim towards the bottom of this range; if they are high (for example, a large man) you could aim towards the top of this range. If the deficit is much below this range then the rate of weight loss will be discouragingly slow. You can now calculate approximately how long it will take you to reach your target weight by deciding how much weight you need to lose and then working out how many weeks this represents if one to two pounds (0.5–1 kg) are lost per week. If your energy deficit is much larger than this suggested range then:

- ■ it is difficult to achieve adequate intakes of vitamins and minerals;
- ■ there will be excessive loss of lean tissue;
- ■ ketosis (see Chapter 5) is increasingly likely.

Sustained moderate energy deficit gives high quality weight loss where a high proportion of the loss is fat. The quality of weight loss also tends to increase with time in those who are overweight – if one maintains the energy deficit, then the rate of weight loss may slow but the proportion that is fat increases.

The body does adapt to starvation and dieting by slowing its metabolism and burning less energy. However, this reduction is modest and is minimised if the diet is a moderate one. Exercise seems to reduce this fall in metabolic rate. Metabolic rate does return to normal after dieting (see Chapter 2).

Losing weight is only half the battle won

The most dispiriting feature of dieting, for both the dieter and therapist, is the tendency to 'relapse'. Even those people who do succeed in losing weight usually regain it in the following months and years (see yo-yo-dieting in Chapter 2). Any weight control programme must offer hope that any weight losses will be maintained once the phase of strict calorie control is over. It must offer a general dietary and lifestyle pattern that favours weight maintenance even without strict calorie counting.

Exercise and weight loss

There are two sides to the energy balance equation, output as well as input can vary. Increased exercise is currently the only practical way of increasing energy output substantially – exercise is important for successful, long-term weight control.

There is little doubt that moderate exercise has general health benefits and there are some obvious effects of increased training on the body, such as:

- improved heart and lung function – we are less breathless after exertion and there is a smaller rise in heart rate;
- increased endurance – we can walk/run further or play/work for longer;
- increased strength;
- increased flexibility – the range of movement is improved.

Several detailed surveys conducted in Britain in recent years have provided shocking evidence of just how inactive and unfit the nation has become. British children walk 20 per cent less than they did just ten years ago and cycle 25 per cent less. Other evidence of declining activity was discussed in Chapter 4. Levels of fitness, strength, flexibility and endurance all decline dramatically as adults go towards middle-age and beyond. These changes are largely the result of declining activity rather than the inevitable consequences of ageing itself, and the trends are already well established in early middle age. People who remain active as they get older, buck these general trends, for example, the fittest 10 per cent of men aged 65–75 are actually fitter than the bottom 10 per cent in the 25–35 age group. The extreme inactivity of many people is making them unable to perform everyday activities in later life, well before the inevitable effects of age itself should. For example:

- many elderly women do not have enough strength in their legs to rise from a chair without using their arms;
- many elderly and even middle-aged people do not have enough shoulder flexibility to allow them to wash their own hair in comfort;
- many middle-aged and elderly people cannot walk at three miles per hour and walking a quarter of a mile unaided is beyond many 70 year olds.

Numerous scientific studies have found that health prospects are better for those who are fit and active and some examples of the demonstrable benefits of regular exercise are given below.

- Active people and those who perform best in scientific 'fitness test' live longer than those who are inactive and unfit.
- Men engaging in vigorous leisure time activities have fewer heart attacks than men who do not. Men with active jobs have fewer heart attacks than those with similar but less active jobs. Exercise increases the amount of 'good cholesterol'–**High Density Lipoproteins (HDL)**–in the blood that protects against heart disease.
- Weight bearing exercise makes bones stronger and reduces the risk of fractures, due to osteoporosis, in later life. Immobility makes bones become thinner and more fragile.
- Regular exercise reduces the risk of strokes.
- Increased activity and fitness have psychological benefits – less depression, anxiety and an increased sense of wellbeing.
- Exercise increases the amount of food we need to eat and so should increase our intake of other nutrients (especially important in the elderly).
- Exercise maintains our ability to perform the activities of daily living in our later years and so maintains morale, self-esteem and quality of life.
- People who are physically fit seem to be protected against the consequences of being overweight or even mildly obese (see Chapter 2).

Aerobic capacity is a scientific measure of fitness which reflects the capacity of the heart and lungs to deliver oxygen to the muscles. In order to get measurable changes in aerobic capacity, then, exercise must be of a certain minimum intensity and duration, for example three, 20-minute sessions each week where heart rate is raised to 70 per cent of its maximum. This is the origin of the maxim that there can be 'no gain without pain'. However, many of the other benefits of exercise accrue even if exercise is only of light to moderate intensity. Activity does not have to be intense and stressful to be beneficial.

Specific benefits of exercise for the dieter

The most obvious way in which exercise could contribute to weight control is by burning off calories. Prolonged bouts of sustainable activity like aerobics, jogging or walking are needed in order to burn off substantial amounts of energy. During such sustainable exercises, the supply of oxygen to the muscles is sufficient for the muscle to produce energy by the normal **aerobic** (oxygen-requiring) processes, hence **aerobic exercise**. It has been argued that unfit and obese people can manage so little aerobic exercise, that its contribution to calorie consumption and weight loss will be negligible. Simple calculations can be done such as, 'in order to burn off one pound of fat tissue you will need to walk briskly for many hours'. However, such calculations seriously underestimate the importance of increased physical activity to weight control, especially if there is an attempt to incorporate more activity into everyday life.

Physical activity levels

Table 6.1 shows how the energy needed to achieve balance and that required to produce a 500 or 1000 calorie deficit rises with the general level of physical activity of the individual. (Remember that **Physical Activity Level, PAL,** is a measure of the overall daily activity and was discussed in Chapter 1). A 10 stone (140 lb/65 kg) woman who is extremely sedentary (PAL 1.3), who is largely housebound, who never walks anywhere and who never participates in active leisure-time pursuits can eat less than 800 calories if she is aiming for a 1000 calorie deficit. This is well below the normal lower limit (say 1200 calories) that most nutritionists think is reasonable to be used in prolonged, unsupervised dieting. However, if this woman raises her physical activity level from the very low level of 1.3 to a still modest 1.5 then she can now consume over 1000 calories per day and still maintain the 1000 calorie deficit. As a rough rule of thumb, it requires about four hours walking per week to raise the PAL by 0.1 points. If this woman raises her activity to the 1.7 level then she achieves a 1000 calorie deficit even when her intake is over 1300 calories per day – a reasonable minimum for prolonged dieting.

Some ideas for raising PAL are suggested later in the chapter, but it will require more than just a weekly aerobics class or game of tennis. To produce a 500 calorie increase in energy expenditure by a single exercise event is time-consuming, for example, several hours walking or nearly two hours of slow jogging. To raise the PAL most effectively, one needs to incorporate more activity into everyday tasks as well as regular participation in some active leisure-time pursuits.

Table 6.1 The energy needs of a 65 kg woman at various Physical Activity Levels (PAL) to achieve energy balance and a 500 or 1000 calorie deficit

	PAL multiple					
	1.0	**1.3**	**1.5**	**1.7**	**2.0**	**2.2**
Calories needed:						
for balance	1375	1788	2063	2338	2750	3025
500 calorie deficit	875	1288	1563	1838	2250	2525
1000 calorie deficit	375	788	1063	1338	1750	2025

The PAL multiple is the figure by which the **Basal Metabolic Rate (BMR)** is multiplied to allow for the energy consumed by the day's physical activity (see Chapter 1).

1.3 represents an extremely inactive person – a largely housebound elderly person or a sedentary office worker who drives everywhere and never takes voluntary exercise.

1.5 represents someone like a teacher who walks around quite a bit whilst they are working.

1.7 a person who walks around quite a bit at work and also takes part in some regular leisure-time physical activity – say, jogs several times a week.

2.0 someone whose job involves a lot of heavy manual work and who probably also takes part in regular vigorous leisure-time pursuits.

2.2+ represents a serious athlete during training.

Note that a brisk 30–40 minute walk would increase the PAL by around 0.1 on that day.

Anaerobic exercise

Exercise not only burns energy directly but can also increase general energy expenditure even when resting because it produces a rise in the Basal Metabolic Rate (BMR). Much of this general increase is due to an increase in the amount of energy-burning muscle tissue in the body. Unused muscles waste (atrophy) whereas well-used muscles get bigger. The most effective exercises for increasing muscle mass are high intensity, short duration activities where the effort involved is close to the maximum, for example, lifting a heavy weight, pushing against a resistance, press ups, jumping, climbing stairs or sprinting. Such exercises are so intense that the oxygen supply to the muscle is insufficient to produce all the energy needed for the intense activity and so the muscle temporarily 'tops up' the energy supply by switching to energy-producing processes that are anaerobic (not requiring oxygen), hence anaerobic exercise. Inactivity reduces BMR because muscle mass falls. BMR falls as adults age because muscles waste and this wasting is largely a consequence of the disuse atrophy that results from inactivity. Anaerobic exercises (weight training) can even produce measurable increases in muscle mass in people in their 80s and 90s.

In their different ways, both aerobic and anaerobic exercises can contribute to weight control. Aerobic exercises can continue for extended periods and so burn up substantial amounts of energy but their effects on muscle mass are modest. Anaerobic exercises are of short duration and so burn up few calories directly but they increase or maintain muscle mass and so raise or maintain resting energy expenditure.

As most people try to lose weight for largely cosmetic reasons, then one other important benefit of exercise for the dieter is its toning effect. People who are fit and active look firmer and better at any given body weight than people who are inactive and flabby.

Exercise helps maintain weight loss

At levels that are achievable by untrained and especially by overweight adults, exercise alone is unlikely to be effective in producing substantial weight loss, it needs to be combined with a reducing diet. It must also be said at this point that in most studies that have looked at the contribution of exercise to weight loss programmes, the conclusion has been that the exercise has led to only a modest increase in weight loss as compared to dieting alone. However, when longer-term outcome has been assessed, the evidence is that an exercise component increases the chances of long-term success. Once people have lost weight and relaxed their diet, they are less likely to regain weight if their programme includes an exercise element; as was said earlier, keeping lost weight off is even more of a challenge than losing it in the first place.

Declining activity is undoubtedly a major cause of the increasing prevalence of obesity. This suggests that being active should help prevent excessive weight gain in the first place; fit and active people do not usually get fat whereas overweight and obese people do tend to be more inactive than lean people. I suggested in Chapter 4 that weight gain and inactivity produce a vicious cycle – not only does inactivity lead to weight gain but weight gain also reduces exercise tolerance which reduces activity still further. In unfit, overweight people, then, initial exercise tolerance will be low and can initially make only a small impact upon energy expenditure, but as conditioning occurs, so tolerance and willingness to exercise increases, leading to a steadily increasing impact upon energy expenditure – a virtuous cycle:

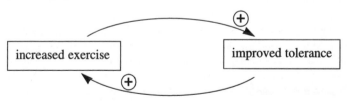

Remember also that only a tiny sustained calorie surplus is required to produce massive long-term weight gain. The relatively small contribution of modest amounts of exercise to energy expenditure look more significant when considered in this context.

Ways of increasing activity and energy expenditure

Be patient. Increase your activity level gradually, especially your participation in any vigorous games or 'workouts'. It can be dangerous to suddenly try to participate in very strenuous activities if you are unfit, overweight and/or no longer young – if you have any doubts or worries (for example chest pains) or if your BMI is over 30 then get professional advice. Sudden, large increases in activity will certainly cause considerable discomfort both during the activity and in the following days of aches and stiffness. If you are unlucky it may cause worse problems such as muscle or joint injuries and very occasionally heart problems or strokes. If you are planning to undertake some formal exercise programme (for example aerobics, 'step' aerobics or weight training) then do this at classes that are supervised by a qualified instructor who should build up your programme gradually and safely.

I would advocate a two-pronged approach to increasing your energy expenditure. Look to increase your activity not just by participating in active leisure-time pursuits but also look for ways of trying to incorporate more activity into everyday living. If exercise is to make a real difference to your Physical Activity Level and your total energy expenditure, then it must be of substantial duration. Have you got the space in your daily schedule to devote enough time to leisure-time exercise to significantly increase your overall activity level? It may be possible to achieve prolonged total periods of activity by an accumulation of short periods of activity incorporated into everyday tasks or during odd moments of dead time during even the busiest day. Some of these may not actually involve any real time costs, for example, it may be quicker to walk rather than to drive short distances in heavy traffic and then find a parking space; it may be quicker to use the stairs than to wait for the lift.

Choose something you enjoy

When considering what leisure-time pursuits to take up or restart, then try to do things that you will enjoy. If you enjoy formal exercise classes or jogging then fine but there are many alternatives. Consider what options are open to you; this will depend upon the local facilities, your capabilities, the time and resources you can afford to devote to them.

Active pursuits should not be in place of a social life but could increase your opportunities for socialising and increase the quality of your life over and above their effects upon your health and weight. If you choose activities that you enjoy and look forward to then it is much more likely that you will keep them up and participate regularly; they will become an integral part of your life – something you do for enjoyment rather than solely for their health and weight control benefits. You may enjoy the intense activity of the squash court, but remember that frequency and duration are more important than intensity – a round of golf (but not if you ride on the golf cart), a game of social tennis or bowls, a hike through the woods can all make useful contributions to boosting your activity level and energy expenditure. Any extra walking or preparation time you spend as a result of your activity can also contribute to increasing your energy expenditure.

Make your everyday life more active

What about incorporating more activity into your everyday life? You can learn a lot about yourself by keeping an activity diary. Break each day up into short time blocks and keep a detailed record of what you do during each time block over a typical working week. Then use this diary to see how you could incorporate more activity into your existing schedule without unduly disrupting your life or committing large blocks of useful time to formal exercise. Remember that the aim is to permanently incorporate these changes into your day so that they become the automatic thing to do. Some examples are given below.

- ■ Can any of the car journeys you make be made by foot or bicycle? In Britain, journeys of less than a mile account for around a third of all car journeys and these short journeys have been increasing rapidly as a proportion of total car journeys. Many of these short journeys could be made on foot or by bicycle – a contribution to the environment as well as the other benefits! When you have to drive, could you park a little way from your destination (even the far side of the parking lot would be a start)? If someone drives you, could you get them to drop you a little way from your destination?

- ■ Could you sometimes use the stairs rather than the lift ? Even if you live or work on a very high floor you could get out two or three floors below and walk the rest of the way.

■ Do you take 'active' steps to minimise your walking? For example, do you ask someone else to bring you a coffee from the canteen or your lunch from the local shop. Do you even minimise the energy expenditure during your leisure-time activities by riding on a golf cart or driving the short distance to the sport's centre?

■ Are there any tasks that are currently done by machine or that you pay someone else to do that you could do for yourself such as car washing, window cleaning, hedge trimming etc? Do you really need to buy yet another labour-saving gadget?

■ Are there any odd moments of 'dead time' in which you could do something active? Could you incorporate a walk into some of your work breaks or do a few exercises while you are waiting for the kids to get ready for bed?

■ Is your garden largely designed to minimise the work required for maintenance? Might you get some pleasure and satisfaction from pottering more and being more ambitious and creative?

■ Would your dog benefit from a regular evening walk? (Driving to the park and allowing it to run around whilst you sit and wait does not count!)

■ Do you spend enough time playing with your children? You all might benefit physically and emotionally from more time actively playing together.

■ How much time do you spend in totally passive activities, especially watching television? The average Briton now watches twice as much television as they did in the 1960s. Many people now spend more time watching television than they do at work or school. How much of this is low quality, habit viewing? If you just switched off the TV during some of this 'low quality' viewing time you would probably be more active and achieve more in your leisure time. Does watching TV encourage inertia and prevent you from doing things and going places that would give you more pleasure and satisfaction? Does watching TV encourage you to snack? By using the video recorder we can fit our quality viewing into time slots of our own choosing rather than fit our other activities around the TV schedule. Remember that studies with obese children found that simply reducing access to sedentary activities like TV and computer games (by a system of persuasion and rewards) was effective in long-term reduction in obesity and was actually more effective than programmes involving strenuous aerobic exercise sessions (see Chapter 4).

■ Does the word holiday conjure up images of resting – lying or sitting around doing nothing but sunbathing, reading or watching TV, punctuated only by frequent bouts of eating and drinking? Might you not get more benefit and pleasure from your holidays if you did some of the more active things you do not normally have time for – playing games with the kids, swimming and other sports, walking, sightseeing on foot?

Table 6.2 The approximate energy costs of various activities expressed as a multiple of Basal Metabolic Rate and as the absolute energy consumption (calories/hour) for a 65 kg woman

BMR multiple	Cals/hour (65 kg woman)	Examples of activities
1.0	60	Lying down – resting*
1.2–1.4	72–84	Sitting – watching TV, reading, writing, playing cards. Standing still.
1.5–1.8	90–108	Sitting – sewing, knitting, driving, playing piano. Standing – peeling vegetables, washing dishes, ironing.
1.9–2.4	114–144	Playing bowls, washing small clothes, playing pool or billiards, hairdressing, dusting.
2.5–3.3	150–180	Dressing and undressing, showering, vacuum cleaning,

		walking at 2–2.5 mph, painting and decorating, operating machine tools.
3.4–4.4	204–264	Mopping floors, general gardening, cleaning windows, table tennis, walking at 2.5–4 mph, bricklaying.
4.5–5.9	270–354	Polishing furniture, chopping wood, heavy gardening, volleyball, energetic dancing, slow jogging, moderate swimming, gentle cycling, heavy labouring work e.g. digging, hoeing, felling trees.
6.0-6.9	360–414	Walking uphill with load, stair climbing, average jogging, soccer, tennis, skiing.

Sustained expenditure above this level is probably beyond most untrained people but is exceeded by trained athletes during training and competition.

*When sleeping the metabolic rate may fall slightly below the BMR.

Data Source: Dietary reference values for food energy and nutrients in the United Kingdom. London: HMSO 1991

Change your attitude to exercise

What I am suggesting is a change of attitude to exercise – the least energy-requiring way of achieving an end should not automatically be regarded as the best option – new labour-saving devices should not necessarily be regarded as an asset if the time saved is then used for totally passive activities like watching TV. Set yourself a time target for increasing the number of minutes during the day when you are going to be more active, include both your formal, leisure-time activities and these extra minutes of incorporated exercise. If you achieve say an hour's extra activity in the day then this might raise your Physical Activity Level by 0.2 points. Table 6.2 gives you some idea of the energy costs of various activities. These values should be taken only as a very approximate guide but they will enable you to get a feel for the amount of extra energy expenditure you have incorporated into your new active day. Remember that frequency and total duration are the priority, not intensity. Remember also that the energy cost of any activity increases with increasing body weight.

The general nature of the recommended diet

As noted in Chapter 5, any diet should have certain utilitarian characteristics that make it a practical proposition for people to use as their diet for life: it should be varied and use food from all the food groups; it should not involve large amounts of extra preparation time; it should use readily available and affordable foods; it should improve long-term health prospects as well as being conducive to weight loss; it should be consistent with the normal cultural eating pattern and be compatible with a normal family diet. A daily energy deficit of 500–1000 calories should achieve steady weight loss without risk of deficiencies, provided that the diet is well constructed and the person is reasonably active.

The diet should be low in fat with perhaps as little as 20–25 per cent of the calories coming from fat during active weight reduction as compared to around 40 per cent in many British and American diets. The bulk of the calories should come from carbohydrates. These carbohydrate calories should predominantly come from starch and those sugars that are naturally present in fruits, vegetables and milk. Sugars that are added to foods during cooking and processing should be minimised during active weight reduction. Intake of dietary fibre should be increased by at least 50 per cent. Apart from the calorie restriction, this general diet structure would be considered a good diet for most adults even if there is no need to lose weight. Even without deliberate calorie restriction, such a diet, when coupled with a reasonably active lifestyle, often produces weight loss *per se* and should certainly prevent weight gain or regain after successful dieting. When weight loss is not required then some relaxation of the sugar and fat restrictions would be expected and acceptable. Such relaxations would be desirable and necessary in rapidly growing children; overenthusiastic restriction of fat and sugar in active rapidly growing children may limit their growth. Children need diets which are nutrient rich and not too energy dilute; inactivity, rather than a fatty/sugary diet, is probably the key to childhood obesity. Overemphasis on healthy eating and fat and sugar restriction may encourage development of eating disorders. It is sometimes difficult to balance the need to establish good eating habits early in life and the need to supply a diet that can support the growth of active youngsters.

Desirable dietary structures

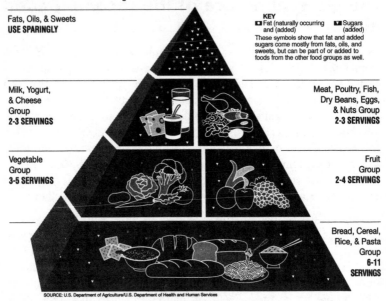

KEY
□ Fat (naturally occurring and (added)   ▼ Sugars (added)
These symbols show that fat and added sugars come mostly from fats, oils, and sweets, but can be part of or added to foods from the other food groups as well.

Fats, Oils, & Sweets
USE SPARINGLY

Milk, Yogurt, & Cheese Group
2-3 SERVINGS

Meat, Poultry, Fish, Dry Beans, Eggs, & Nuts Group
2-3 SERVINGS

Vegetable Group
3-5 SERVINGS

Fruit Group
2-4 SERVINGS

Bread, Cereal, Rice, & Pasta Group
6-11 SERVINGS

SOURCE: U.S. Department of Agriculture/U.S. Department of Health and Human Services

6.1   The American Food Guide Pyramid

Figures 6.1 and 6.2 show respectively the American Food Guide Pyramid and the British Food Guide Plate. These are visual indicators of the type of dietary structure that is considered desirable upon general health grounds for all adults and older children. If coupled with rigorous attempts to minimise consumption of fats and added sugar then this diet structure should achieve the compositional objectives for dieters that I have listed. Although they use very different images, these guides are indicating essentially the same sort of diet:

> ■ Starchy cereals and potatoes should provide the bulk of the daily calories. These foods provide the bulk of calories in most peasant diets but their contribution to British and American diets have declined dramatically in this century. In

their natural state, these foods are high in starch and fibre but contain almost no fat. Although they provide energy as starch they have a relatively low energy concentration and produce a bulky diet. One should preferentially choose the unrefined, whole grain foods within the group which have their dietary fibre and natural nutrients left in. Dieters must minimise use of foods in this category to which large amounts of fat and/or sugar have been added, for example, fried potatoes, cookies, cakes, fried rice, over-sweetened breakfast cereals.

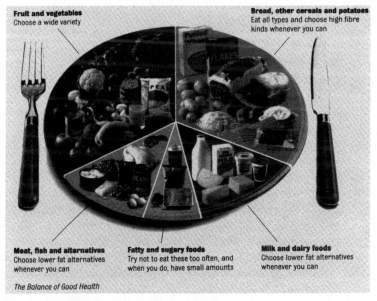

Fruit and vegetables
Choose a wide variety

Bread, other cereals and potatoes
Eat all types and choose high fibre kinds whenever you can

Meat, fish and alternatives
Choose lower fat alternatives whenever you can

Fatty and sugary foods
Try not to eat these too often, and when you do, have small amounts

Milk and dairy foods
Choose lower fat alternatives whenever you can

The Balance of Good Health

6.2 The British Food Guide Plate
Source: Health Education Authority, The Balance of Good Health

■ The diet should contain large and varied amounts of fruits and vegetables. These foods are rich in many essential nutrients. In their natural state, they are almost always low in calories, practically devoid of fat (avocados are a rare exception), and have good amounts of dietary fibre. They have a very low energy concentration and so even if large weights are eaten this represents few calories (see p.72 Chapter 4). There is evidence that simply eating more of these foods in an unrestrained situation may lead to a reduction in the proportion of calories that are derived from fat. Dieters should minimise use of fruits and vegetables which have had fat and sugar added to them, for example fried vegetables, vegetables mashed or topped with butter or margarine, fruits canned in syrup, fatty or oily dressings. Most vegetables and fruits can be eaten fairly freely provided no sugar or fat has been added to them, for example:

- green leafy vegetables;
- most salad vegetables (not avocado);
- most citrus and other fruits;
- most root vegetables (potatoes should be treated like starchy cereals).

■ A good and adequate diet needs foods from the meat and milk groups (these groups include beans, peas, nuts, vegetarian milks and modern meat substitutes) because these foods are a major source of several important nutrients such as protein, calcium, iron, vitamin B12 and riboflavin. However, because they are very palatable, we tend to consume more of them than is good for us, and so moderating their use is desirable for improving our health prospects. These foods provide some 40–50 per cent of the fat and saturated fat in our diets. Much of this fat can be avoided by moderating use of these foods and by choosing the low fat options within these groups, such as:

- grilled (broiled), baked or boiled lean meat, skinned poultry and white fish;
- low fat milk, cheese and yoghurt;
- dried peas and beans.

■ The remaining fatty and sugary foods provide many calories in the form of fats and sugars but few nutrients. They need to be ruthlessly controlled during active attempts at weight reduction.

Fat appears to be more fattening than sugar and other carbohydrates (see Chapters 3 and 4). During active weight reduction, intake of both fatty and sugary foods should be minimised but fat reduction should be the priority for weight loss and probably would be the nutrition priority on other health grounds as well. Some practical ways of reducing fat and calorie intake are suggested in Table 6.3.

Artificial sweeteners, reduced fat foods and fat substitutes

Artificial sweetners

At first sight, artificial sweeteners would seem like a great asset to dieters. If a glass of regular cola is replaced by diet cola then this saves about 75 calories, if 10 daily spoonfuls of sugar are replaced by a calorie-free sweetener then this saves about 200 calories. As sugars make up 15-20 per cent of our total calorie intake then they seem to offer great scope for relatively simple and painless calorie reduction. However, the massive increase in the use of artificial sweeteners in recent decades has not been accompanied by corresponding reductions in sugar use and it has actually coincided with a large increase in people's fatness.

In theory, saccharin, aspartame and other sweeteners save us from consuming billions of sugar calories each year, calorie savings that are probably equivalent to several pounds of prevented weight gain for every Briton and American. Calorie-free sweeteners can save 'empty' sugar calories but they will not have the satiating effect of sugar and so without conscious calorie control we will tend to replace the lost calories with other food. When people introduce sugar substitutes into their everyday diets then the evidence is that they replace the lost sugar calories with other food providing mixed calories, and so the proportion of their energy that they derive from fat actually increases. Sugar substitutes may be useful as part of a calorie-controlled diet but paradoxically if just introduced as a single easy measure into an unregulated diet they may actually favour increased consumption of fat calories and perhaps even weight gain.

Reduced fat products

Similar arguments to those above suggest that if reduced fat products are used, then if they are replaced by mixed calories, the proportion of calories derived from fat should decline. As fat calories are poorly detected by our hunger control mechanisms then one might expect this to lead to better regulation of body weight in its own right. There is evidence that stringent dietary fat reduction leads to reduced overall energy intake and weight loss even without conscious calorie restriction.

Fat restriction, even without deliberate energy restriction, may favour weight loss and should certainly limit weight gain and regain.

Reduced fat products may make a useful contribution to reducing overall fat intake. There may, however, well be more effective and certainly cheaper ways of reducing fat intake i.e. by choosing more of the foods that are naturally low in fat or avoiding the visible fat in meals. Reduced fat foods are sometimes an expensive way of achieving rather modest reductions in fat.

Fat substitutes

What about fat substitutes? Some synthetic fats give food the beneficial effects of fat upon palatability but are either not digested and absorbed from the gut or have a lower energy yield than natural fats. One of these products is a synthetic fat called olestra which is not digested and goes through the gut unaltered. It has gained approval in the US for limited use in savoury snack foods like potato crisps/chips but is not permitted in Europe. There are a number of short-term problems with such products and many scientists have serious concerns about the long-term effects of regularly eating foods containing such products. In the short-term, they can cause problems because of the entry of indigestible fatty material into the large bowel resulting in diarrhoea, bowel urgency, anal leakage, abdominal cramps, greasy staining of toilets and underwear. They also reduce the absorption of fat soluble substances including fat soluble vitamins and cholesterol. In the USA, foods containing olestra have to be fortified with fat soluble vitamins to compensate for their reduced absorption although there may well be other, unknown but beneficial fat soluble substances in foods. Olestra is currently restricted to use in savoury snacks in the USA on the grounds that these foods are not usually eaten with meals and so the olestra will not interfere with the absorption of vitamins in normal meals. Compounds like olestra are being promoted as potentially able to replace up to 30 g of fat per day in the diet (270 calories) but many doubts remain:

■ Will the use of these compounds really reduce overall fat consumption or will they simply be additions to the current diet? Might they even encourage our fat preference and cause us to eat more fatty foods?

■ Are the immediate effects upon bowel function and nutrient absorption acceptable for a deliberate food additive or can they be eliminated? As one American pressure group puts it 'would you feed this product to your pet dog?'

■ What are the long-term consequences of the change in the environment in the large bowel? We are encouraged to believe that differences in the fat and/or fibre content of the diet can substantially affect our susceptibility to diseases like bowel cancer, because they produce changes in the bowel environment. Here we have substances that will undeniably produce radical alterations in the bowel environment; are we to trust that in 10 or 20 years some unforeseen consequences of this change will not start to emerge?

Other ways of losing fat and calories from your diet

A sample page from a completed food diary

Time	Description of food or drink	Amount of serving e.g. cup, slice, spoonful	Leftover
07:30	Weetabix	2 biscuits	
	semi-skimmed milk	1 cup	
	sugar	1 teaspoon	
	coffee with semi-skimmed milk, no sugar	2 cups	
	wholemeal toast	2 slices large loaf	
	butter	medium layers	
	marmalade	2 tspns	
10.30	coffee with whole milk, no sugar	1 mug	

	chocolate digestive biscuits	2
12:30	whole meal bread	3 slices large loaf
	butter	thinly spread
	ham	3 thin slices
	tomato	1 medium
	cucumber	6 slices
	banana	1 medium
	apple	1 medium
15:30	tea with whole milk, no sugar	1 mug
17:30	coffee with semi-skimmed milk	1 mug
18:30	chicken breast (fried in olive oil with skin, no bone)	1
	Jacket potato	1 large
	butter	1 tsp
	baked beans	2 tbsp
	orange	1 large
	dry white wine	2 glasses
	coffee with semi-skimmed milk, no sugar	2 cups
20:00	unsweetened orange juice	1 glass
21:00	lager beer	1 large can
23:00	drinking chocolate (made with semi-skimmed milk)	1 mug

Source: Webb, GP and Copeman, J 1996 *The nutrition of older adults* London: Arnold p.157.

The first stage in devising a personalised diet is to find out what your current diet is like. Keep a detailed record of everything that you eat and drink for a week (see pp.137–8). Remember that you are trying to get an accurate picture of your usual diet. If you cheat and modify your diet during this period then you are only cheating yourself. Once you have completed this diary, look to see whether it complies with the general pattern suggested by the pyramid and plate in Figures 6.1 and 6.2. Is it based upon starchy cereals and potatoes? Does it contain at least five portions of fruits and vegetables each day (excluding potatoes)? Or, is it heavily biased towards the foods of the meat and milk groups? Does it make liberal use of calorie-rich but nutrient depleted fatty and sugary foods? Look to modify the meals that you normally consume so that the overall diet starts to take on the shape suggested by Figures 6.1 and 6.2.

Fat, added sugar and alcohol currently provide more than 55 per cent of the total calories in average diets of Britons and Americans. It is from these sources that one should be looking to make the bulk of the calorie reductions. A woman eating around 2000 calories per day, may be eating as much as 90 g of fat each day. Cutting this fat consumption in half would result in a direct saving of up to 400 calories and if coupled with a moderate increase in activity could bring her an energy deficit in the target range (500–1000 calories).

Look for obvious sources of added sugar and fat in your diet, for example, regular consumption of fatty or sugary snacks and drinks. These should be replaced by low calorie foods such as fruit, pieces of raw vegetables and sugar-free drinks. If appropriate, moderate your alcohol intake – no more than a small glass or two of dry wine per day for a dieting woman. Look for other sources of fat in your diet than can be replaced or modified so as to save fat. Here are some tips for fat and calorie reduction:

- avoid cakes, pastries, candies and chocolate;
- buy leaner cuts of meat and use more white fish;
- remove all visible fat from meat and skim off fat when cooking meat dishes;
- remove the skin from poultry and pork;
- limit use of oily nuts, seeds and peanut butter;
- avoid fish canned in oil, choose those canned in water or tomato sauce;

- avoid high fat meat and fish products such as sausages, pies, burgers, and anything, animal or vegetable, that is coated in batter, crispy crumbs or has a pastry case;
- replace full fat milk with low fat milk – skimmed milk is virtually fat-free;
- avoid products made with whole milk such as shakes;
- minimise use of spreading fats like butter and margarine –low fat spreads may help but not if you use more. Try some sandwiches without any fat spread, you may not miss them if the bread is fresh and the filling is moist;
- moderate use of cheese, and replace ordinary cheese with low fat cheeses or perhaps with lean cooked meats like lean ham, chicken or turkey, avoid full fat soft cheeses;
- minimise use of fatty or oily dressings or toppings for salads, vegetables and baked potatoes;
- minimise the use of sugar at the table and in cooking;
- avoid cream or cream substitutes made with vegetable oil;
- avoid sugary drinks;
- minimise use of cooking fats and oils – bake, boil or grill (broil) rather than fry, or try using a fat-free frying pan;
- avoid sauces and gravies which are high in fat, for example cheese sauce and those made with meat juices;
- avoid crisps (potato chips) and similar savoury snacks;
- restrict your alcoholic intake to small amounts of dry wine and spirits with sugar-free mixers – note that alcohol itself provides calories;
- if you use a lot of prepared foods or meals then choose low fat versions or replace with reduced-fat home cooked meals;
- the fat in oily fish like mackerel, herring and sardines may have beneficial effects and increases in fatty fish consumption is generally recommended, however, this fat is still high in calories and must be eaten in moderation during active weight reduction.

Table 6.3 gives some examples of the fat and calorie savings that can be achieved by modifying your existing choices. Remember that these fat and/or calorie reductions apply only if they are not replaced by more of something else!

Table 6.3 Examples of typical fat and calorie reductions. Portion sizes are 'typical usual' portions and portions of replacements are matched unless otherwise indicated

Approx metric conversions	28 g = 1 oz
	50 g = 1.75 oz
	100 g = 3.5 oz
	150 g = 5.5 oz
	200 g = 7 oz

Food *Alternative*	Fat (g) *– saving*	Energy (kcal) *– saving*
pint whole milk (UK)	20.5	375
semi skimmed	*-11*	*-114*
skimmed	*-20*	*-188*
butter/margarine (10 g)	8	74
low fat spread	*-4*	*-37*
very low fat	*-5.5*	*-47*
no spread	*-8*	*-74*
cheddar cheese (60 g)	20.5	248
reduced fat	*-11.5*	*-92*
lean ham	*-17.5*	*-176*
'Speciality' burger with cheese	32.5	560
'Quarter pounder'	*-12*	*-150*
regular hamburger	*-23*	*-297*
French fries (large)	21.5	400
regular	*-4.5*	*-80*
small	*-9.5*	*-180*
milk shake (fast food outlet)	10.5	390
regular cola	*-10.5*	*-246*
diet cola	*-10.5*	*-389*
two teaspoons of sugar	0	40
saccharin or *aspartame*	*0*	*-40*

double cream on dessert	17	157
single cream	*-10*	*-88*
no cream	*-17*	*-157*
fried egg	8.5	107
boiled/poached	*-2*	*-19*
quiche, cheese (100 g)	22.5	314
ham and tomato sandwich *(no fat spread)*	*-19*	*-198*
spaghetti (150 g) + bolognese (140 g)	16.5	351
only 70 g bolognese	*-7.5*	*-98*
70 g sauce (lean mince)	*-11.5*	*-143*
70 g tomato sauce	*-12*	*-135*
mayonnaise (20 g)	15	138
reduced calorie	-9.5	-80
vinegar-only dressing	-15	-138
tablespoon oil/vinegar	8	70
vinegar only	*-8*	*-70*
fried battered cod (100 g)	10.5	199
boiled/baked/grilled cod	*-9*	*-104*
battered fried chicken leg	25.5	431
eat meat only	*-16.5*	*-235*
roast chicken leg & skin	15.5	264
eat meat only	*-7.5*	*-83*
egg fried rice (190 g)	20	395
boiled rice	*-19.5*	*-162*
cauliflower cheese (165 g)	11.5	173
cauliflower only	*-11.5*	*-158*
chips (fried potatoes) (200g)		
thin 'fast-food' fries	31	560
English fish & chip shop	*-6*	*-82*
chips (steak fries) homemade *(large and well drained)*	*-17.5*	*-182*
oven chips/fries	*-22.5*	*-236*

mashed potato	*-22.5*	*-352*
boiled potatoes	*-31*	*-416*
potato crisps (30 g packet)	11	160
low fat crisps	*-6.5*	*-23*
one banana	*-10.5*	*-97*
whole milk fruit yoghurt (150 g)	4	158
low fat fruit yoghurt	*-3*	*-23*
low calorie & low fat	*-4*	*-96*
chocolate bar	12.5	287
one apple	*-12.5*	*-245*
2 half-covered chocolate biscuits	7	148
2 plain sweet	*-1*	*-7*
one banana	*-7*	*-85*
slice pizza (160 g)	19.5	320
Baked potato +	*-18.5*	*-109*
(100 g) baked beans		
half pint beer	0	126
glass sweet wine	*-*	*-19*
dry wine	*-*	*-51*
tuna canned in oil (100 g)	8	197
(drained)		
canned water/brine	*-7.5*	*-70*
peanuts roasted (30 g)	16	181
dry roasted	*-1*	*-4*
one banana	*-15.5*	*-118*
fruit pie (120g)	9.5	223
fresh fruit salad	*-9.5*	*-158*
ice cream dairy (75 g)	7.5	146
low calorie	*-2*	*-57*
one apple	*-7.5*	*-104*
Danish pastry	17.5	374
banana	*-17.5*	*-311*

cream cheese (30 g)	14	132
low fat	-7	-70
low fat cottage cheese	-13.5	-108
slice cheesecake (100 g)	10.5	242
banana	*-10*	*-179*
meat pie (165 g)	35	523
(pastry top and bottom)		
pastry top only	*-5*	*-52*
minced beef stewed onion (165 g)	24	317
with extra lean mince	*-12.5*	*-101*
grilled rump/butt steak (155 g)	19	338
(with fat)		
fat removed	*-9.5*	*-85*

Could fat and sugar restriction cause nutrient deficiencies?

Dieting reduces food intake and so it is a potential threat to the adequacy of nutrient intakes. If you eat less of your normal diet then the intake of all nutrients and of fibre will also be reduced. If you cut your portion sizes by 40 per cent then you cut your intake of nutrients and fibre by 40 per cent. This could precipitate deficiencies, increase the risk of constipation and would also be a very noticeable reduction in the total amount of food you eat. However, the diet that has been recommended here should give you more nutrients and more volume of food for every calorie. It should produce a diet that is bulky and richer in fibre and essential nutrients than many current diets.

Added sugars and alcoholic drinks provide lots of calories but few nutrients so reducing them removes energy but has little effect on nutrient intakes. Fat is the most concentrated form of dietary energy but it is also a source of the fat soluble vitamins and the essential fatty acids. In practice, however, even very substantial reductions in fat intake do not threaten our adequacy for these nutrients. The fat that remains, even in low fat diets in the UK and USA would contain adequate amounts of most of these nutrients and several additional factors that also contribute to minimising this risk are listed below.

- Vitamin A is dietetically the most important fat soluble vitamin. Vitamin A itself, **retinol**, can only be obtained from animal foods and is dissolved in the fat. However, we can convert **ß-carotene** found in green, red and yellow fruits and vegetables into retinol, so producing an alternative source of vitamin A. Low fat diets, that are high in fruits and vegetables, may well contain more vitamin A than your current diet. Some foods, for example, low fat milk, low fat spreads, margarine, and some breakfast cereals may be fortified with vitamins including vitamins A and D.

- Dietary vitamin D also comes from fatty animal foods. Vegetables, lean meat and skimmed milk have no vitamin D (unless it has been fortified by added vitamins). However, for most adults, except those who are housebound, the principal source of vitamin D is from sunlight rather than the diet. Those British people who are never exposed to sunlight, such as elderly housebound people, cannot get enough from their diets anyway and need supplements (note that more foods are supplemented with vitamin D in the USA, including milk).

- Deficiencies of vitamins E and K are unlikely to occur and, for vitamin E, requirement is probably reduced if fat intake is reduced.

- Our requirement for essential fatty acids is very small and our fat tissue contains large stores of them. Even very low fat diets, lower than is likely in the USA or UK, will contain the small amounts of these fatty acids that we require. It has proved very difficult to induce essential fatty acid deficiencies in adult human volunteers even when eating diets deliberately designed to be low in these fatty acids for many months.

Animal foods normally make a major contribution to our intakes of several other important nutrients such as calcium, iron, protein, riboflavin and B12 but these are water soluble substances that are concentrated in the lean part of meat and the fat-free part of milk.

Diet compliance and behaviour modification

I suggested earlier that it is not particularly difficult for someone with a basic knowledge of food and nutrition to design a weight loss plan that will work if followed diligently. The major difficulty is in sticking to this plan for the weeks or months that may be necessary to reach one's target weight. Many people find that joining a group like Weightwatchers may help them to maintain their motivation over the weeks and months of dieting. Some of these groups offer a variety of services such as group exercise sessions, home exercise plans, motivational sessions, regular weigh-ins, as well as diet plans and dietary advice. These are often commercial ventures but many, like Weightwatchers, are reputable and offer a valuable and honest service. There are many, however, which are less scrupulous and their sole aim seems to be to lighten our pockets rather than our bodies. The criteria in Chapter 5 may help you to judge competing groups.

Behaviour therapy

One technique that has been widely used to help people stick to a weight loss plan is behaviour modification or **behaviour therapy**. This method evolved from the belief that the feeding behaviour of obese people was abnormal and so was geared towards normalising their feeding behaviour or minimising the consequences of their abnormal behaviour. Lean people were believed to control their food intake largely in response to their internal physiological hunger mechanisms, whereas obese people were more responsive to external, non-physiological influences resulting in poor control. External factors are things such as the time of day, the palatability of food; ease of access to food; sight and smell of food; and, emotional state. The notion that the eating behaviours of lean and obese people are different has become unfashionable but behaviour therapy remains a widely used tool in obesity treatment and readers may find elements of it useful in helping them to stick to their own weight loss programme. Help from a trained behaviour therapist would clearly be necessary to apply this technique fully and most effectively.

Any behaviour is seen as being triggered by certain cues. If the consequence of a behaviour is pleasant then this acts as a reward (positive reinforcement) and this encourages repetition and learning of this behaviour. If the consequence of a behaviour is unpleasant then this punishment (negative reinforcement) discourages its repetition:

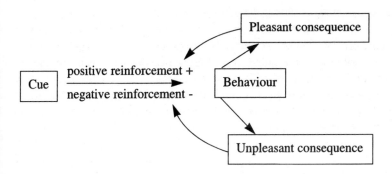

The first step in behaviour therapy is to identify some of the cues that trigger inappropriate eating behaviour by keeping a detailed food diary that would have details not only of what and how much you eat but also:

- when and where you eat;
- the circumstances of eating, for example who you were with, whether you were doing something else at the time, such as reading or watching television;
- your mood at the time – worried, depressed, happy.

From this diary one would then try to identify some of the cues that trigger inappropriate eating so that you can either eliminate them or modify them. The list below gives some of the tips that are used in behaviour therapy to help people minimise their exposure to inappropriate eating cues.

- Shop for food when you have just eaten and are not hungry.
- Make a shopping list and only buy foods on the list.
- Only take enough money for foods on the list.
- As far as possible limit your buying of high calorie/fat foods, for example, could other family members buy and store their own sweets and high calorie snacks?
- Don't buy ready-to-eat foods for immediate consumption, for example, from vending machines but do carry appropriate low calorie/fat snacks with you.
- Avoid food programmes on television.

- Make high calorie/fat snacks less accessible so that eating them has to be a premeditated act rather than something that can be done almost subconsciously – put them on a high shelf or in a locked cupboard.
- Don't put serving dishes on the table, allocate portions onto the plate before sitting at the table.
- Use smaller plates and utensils – this makes small portions less obvious.
- Don't keep leftovers and encourage other family members to dispose of their own leftovers at the end of the meal.
- Don't accept food from others.
- Always eat food in the same designated places and don't do anything else whilst you are eating, for example, watch TV or read.
- Try to avoid boredom as this may be a trigger for eating.

One should also consider ways of increasing cues or making it easier to do appropriate behaviours, for example:

- keep shoes for walking and equipment for active pursuits in view and readily accessible;
- keep low calorie snacks prepared and in a prominent position in the refrigerator;
- take the trouble to prepare permitted foods attractively.

Behaviour therapists often also recommend that their clients modify or control eating behaviour itself, for example, by:

- slowing down the eating process by using smaller utensils, chewing food thoroughly, pausing between mouthfuls, adding a two- to three-minute gap in the middle of the meal;
- always using utensils and not fingers;
- leaving some food on the plate at the end of the meal;
- always eating with other family members.

Therapists encourage their clients to devise a system of rewards for appropriate eating or exercise behaviours or for achieving designated goals. These rewards can take the form of non-food treats ('active' treats would be ideal), praise from other family members or even the use of stickers or stars as used in schools.

When one looks at the cue-behaviour-reinforcement model shown earlier, then some form of negative reinforcement for inappropriate behaviour would seem like a logical inclusion in a behaviour therapy programme. However, most therapists avoid the use of active punishment in their schemes – clients are encouraged to eat with others and ask them to praise and encourage appropriate behaviour but to pointedly ignore inappropriate behaviour and simply withhold praise. Scolding is seen as attention-giving and thus a form of reward whereas the withholding of attention is seen as punishment. In the past, some behaviour therapists have used punishment as an active part of their programme – so-called aversion therapy. Patients were shown images of problem foods followed by painful electric shocks or some other unpleasant image in the hope that they would learn to associate these foods with unpleasant sensations and so avoid them!

Catastrophising

Clients are encouraged to set realistic and achievable goals and to focus on their achievements rather than occasional lapses. It is all too easy after several weeks of steady progress to exaggerate the significance of a relatively minor lapse, lose heart and abandon the effort – so-called **catastrophising**. Over an extended programme one must expect occasional lapses but provided that they really are occasional then you should put them behind you, not attempt to compensate by missing subsequent meals and realise that their impact upon your long-term progress will be modest. They are likely to slow your current progress rather than undo the achievements of several previous weeks – just as it takes a deficit of 7000 calories to lose 1 kg (2 pounds) of fat tissue, so it takes much more than 7000 surplus calories to undo the loss 1 kg of fat tissue c.f. the 250 calories in the average chocolate bar! Clients are encouraged not to miss meals and thus to create situations of deprivation and extreme hunger that are likely to encourage lapses. Foreseeable occasions when lapses are likely to occur – parties and dining out – should be planned for by saving some calories from preceding meals and by planning one's eating at the event to maximise enjoyment but minimise the damage to one's calorie control, the consumption of a low calorie snack prior to a party is sometimes suggested.

Hypnotherapy

Some therapists employ hypnosis in order to help patients stick to their weight loss programme. It is not an alternative to the diet and exercise programme suggested in this chapter but a means of trying to improve patients' compliance.

Conclusions

■ You are probably the best person to devise the most appropriate weight loss programme for you.

■ The success or failure of your weight loss programme is largely in your hands.

■ There are no short cuts or easy ways of losing lots of weight. You will need to keep your calorie intake below your expenditure for a substantial period of time and this will be difficult and uncomfortable.

■ Increasing activity is very important for preventing excess weight gain (particularly in children) and for preventing weight regain after successful dieting. The contribution of exercise to weight loss during dieting may be modest but it will probably help to reduce losses of lean tissue during weight reduction.

■ Ideally, activity should be increased not only by increased participation in active leisure-time pursuits but also by incorporating more activity into one's everyday schedule.

■ Reducing fat intake is the priority when devising a low calorie reducing diet.

■ Many suggestions for increasing activity and reducing fat intake are suggested in the chapter.

7 | ALTERNATIVES TO DIET AND EXERCISE

Scope of the chapter

In this chapter I will very briefly review the anti-obesity drugs that are currently in use and those that are being tested and developed for possible future use. I will also briefly discuss some of the surgical treatments that may be used to treat severe obesity. I will suggest that these are not really alternatives to diet and exercise but ways of improving compliance with diet and exercise programmes.

Anti-obesity drugs

The idea of a pill to cure obesity is a very attractive one both for chronically overweight people and for the shareholders of drug companies. Drug companies around the world spend many millions of pounds/dollars each year working on a wide variety of potential anti-obesity drugs. All I can do in a book like this is to discuss the few anti-obesity drugs currently in use and outline some of the newer approaches to drug therapy of obesity that are being researched. I cannot hope to discuss the merits and disadvantages of each drug under investigation but I would first offer some general words of caution:

■ All effective drugs have potential side-effects and many carry the risk of producing serious, even fatal side-effects in some individuals. The benefits of using a drug have to be substantial enough to outweigh its risks. Any risks are greatly magnified if drugs are misused – if recommended doses or duration of use are exceeded, if the drug is used in inappropriate circumstances, or if used without professional guidance and monitoring. Some anti-obesity drugs have well-documented side-effects that have caused fatalities in some takers. Their use may be justifiable to help people with severe and intractable obesity, where the health risks of the obesity are high, but not for people whose overweight or mild obesity poses much less risk to their health. In some cases physicians have prescribed them to patients who are not even overweight.

■ Many of the drugs have very limited or dubious effectiveness. All of them will still require a substantial commitment from the taker to be properly effective. You cannot hope to just let the drug do all the work. Remember also that even if drugs help you to lose some weight then eventually you will have to keep off any lost weight without the aid of your chemical crutch. Drugs may make it less painful for patients to stick to their diet by, for example, reducing hunger but they will only work if the patient really does stick to the diet.

■ Will drugs provide a long-term solution to a problem that has its origins in an inappropriate and unhealthy lifestyle? Should we not be focusing our efforts upon the causes rather than trying to find pharmaceutical palliatives with all of their attendant problems and risks?

Drugs that increase the actions of noradrenaline in the brain

Noradrenaline (norepinephrine) acts as a nerve transmitter in the brain where its actions result in an anorectic effect (reduced hunger and food intake) coupled with a stimulation of the sympathetic nervous system – the part of the nervous system responsible for 'flight and fight' or stress responses. Amphetamine increases the actions of this nerve transmitter and was the first anorectic drug to be widely used in obesity treatment. Amphetamine also increases the activity of the nerve transmitter dopamine, which acts as a brain stimulant and produces euphoria. Derivatives of amphetamine have been developed with less of the potentially addictive euphoric (dopamine) effect whilst maintaining the anorectic (noradrenaline) effect. These modified amphetamines have been widely used in America although not elsewhere. These drugs seem to produce only very modest amounts of extra weight loss as compared to placebos. Even this modest effect seems to be confined to the first few weeks of treatment and continued used much beyond the first month does not seem to produce further benefits. Removal of the drug normally leads to rapid regain of the lost weight. This combination of poor long-term effectiveness and the potential for addiction is why the US authorities only permit weight-reducing drugs to be used for a maximum of 12 weeks.

Drugs that increase the actions of 5-HT (serotonin) in the brain

When the nerve transmitter **5-HT (serotonin)** is injected into the brains of animals it decreases feeding, and some anti-obesity drugs work by increasing the actions of this nerve transmitter in the brain. These drugs produce an anorectic effect but without the potentially addictive stimulant effects of the amphetamines or the stimulation of the sympathetic nervous system. Their effect on hunger is also subtly different from that of the amphetamines – rather than reducing the desire to eat as the amphetamines do, they make users feel full earlier and so cause them to stop eating after a smaller intake of food than usual. The compounds **fenfluramine** and the closely related **dexfenfluramine** act in this way. These drugs have been widely used in Europe, fenfluramine has been around for over thirty years and dexfenfluramine for over a decade and tens of millions of people have been treated with them (over 60,000 in Britain in 1996). In Europe, they have been used in long-term trials lasting for a year with some encouraging results. For example, in a year-long trial comparing the effects of dexfenfluramine plus diet versus diet plus placebo, the drug group achieved 30 per cent of the required weight loss compared to 20 per cent in the non-drug group. In 1996, dexfenfluramine was controversially approved for use as a weight-reducing drug in the USA, the first diet pill to receive FDA approval for 20 years.

One rare, but widely accepted, side-effect of these drugs seems to be a potentially fatal lung condition called pulmonary hypertension. There are also suggestions from studies with laboratory animals that they may damage some of the nerve cells in the brain that use 5-HT (serotonin) as a nerve transmitter. In the summer of 1997, new research in the USA suggested that disturbingly high numbers of women taking these drugs had developed problems with their heart valves – a problem that is normally very rare. The FDA in America has since withdrawn the drugs and the French manufacturers have now withdrawn these drugs from the market worldwide 'as a precautionary measure'. The British Royal College of Physicians withdrew its previous recommendation that these drugs could be used as a last resort to treat severe obesity. The withdrawal of these drugs leaves the cupboard pretty bare of currently available, weight-reducing drugs that have any demonstrated effectiveness for more than a short period. Their withdrawal after such wide and prolonged use also demonstrates the difficulty of ensuring that such drugs are safe – a good reason to be cautious about the use of any new anti-obesity drug in all but the most extreme cases. Certainly, all such drug use needs to be very strictly regulated and carefully monitored.

A drug called **sibutramine** has recently been developed which has dual action on both the noradrenaline (norepinephrine) and the 5-HT (serotonin) systems. Combined use of drugs working via each of these routes (half the normal doses of each) had previously been shown to be as effective as single drugs but to produce less side-effects. Its approval from the FDA for use in America is widely believed to be imminent.

Thermogenic agents

Thermogenic (heat-generating) drugs, stimulate metabolism and 'burn off' extra calories. A number of agents are effective in stimulating metabolic rate but their severe and sometimes fatal side-effects render them unusable as weight control agents. A chemical called dinitrophenol was seen to cause weight loss amongst munitions workers in the First World War. For a while it was used as a weight control agent until the full extent of the side-effects, including some fatalities, became apparent. Thyroid hormones also cause an acceleration of metabolism and weight loss but, once again, side-effects make them unsuitable for weight control use.

More recent research in this area has focused upon compounds that might specifically stimulate heat generation in **brown fat** – the tissue known to be important as a heat-generating tissue in small mammals and human babies (see Chapter 3). This tissue is now known to respond to the nerve transmitter noradrenaline via a receptor that is different from that found on most other noradrenaline sensitive cells – the **ß$_3$-adrenoreceptor**. Drugs that specifically stimulate this receptor should stimulate heat production in brown fat but have few unwanted effects upon other tissues. Several ß$_3$ adrenoreceptor stimulants have been produced and have given encouraging results in some trials with rats, although early results with humans are much less encouraging. This could be because:

- the amount of brown fat in adult humans is small compared to rats who need it to keep warm;
- the drugs so far produced fit the rat's ß3-adrenoreceptor much better than the human one.

A specific stimulator of the human ß3-adrenoreceptor has recently been announced. One hope is that it might not just stimulate existing receptors on brown fat but also perhaps stimulate the production of more brown fat cells. Despite more than two decades of intensive searching for safe and effective thermogenic agents, any prospect of one reaching the market in the next few years seems remote and there must be serious doubts about whether this approach will bear any fruit in the foreseeable future.

Drugs that interfere with digestion/ absorption

Several drugs have been developed that inhibit the enzyme **lipase** which is responsible for fat digestion within the gut (for example, **orlistat**). Potential problems with these types of compounds would be similar to those discussed in the previous chapter for non-digestible fat substitutes like olestra.

Note also under this heading the use of some substances that would be classified as food additives/supplements rather than drugs, for example:

- fat substitutes and artificial sweeteners (see Chapter 6);
- bulking agents like fibre supplements and some water holding gels that may help to produce satiety.

A product which is made from the powdered shells of shellfish, such as prawns, shrimps and crabs has recently been marketed as an anti-obesity agent. It is said to bind fat in the gut and so reduce its digestion and absorption. The claims of this compound are speculative and, of course, some of the potential problems of fat substitutes would also apply to this compound.

Cholecystokinin

As discussed in Chapter 3, **cholecystokinin (CCK)** is a hormone released from the gut when food is present in it. This hormone stimulates the release of bile and pancreatic juice into the gut to aid digestion. It also stimulates nerve endings in the gut that signal fullness to the brain's appestat. Injections of CCK in animals reduces appetite. A compound has now been produced that mimics the actions of CCK and works when given orally. It suppresses appetite very effectively in laboratory animals. It is still in the developmental stage and, even if things go well, it is likely to be some years before it becomes available for human use.

CCK is also a nerve transmitter in the brain. Injections of CCK into the brains of animals suppresses appetite and reduces feeding. A chemical called **butabindide** was recently shown to increase the actions of CCK in the brains of experimental animals by blocking the enzymes that normally break down CCK, so reducing food intake and producing weight loss.

What about leptin?

As was discussed at length in Chapter 3, leptin is the satiety hormone produced in fat cells that signals the brain's appestat to reduce hunger and food intake and increase energy expenditure. Leptin injections are very effective in reducing the obesity of genetically obese, ob/ob mice. However, their obesity is caused by leptin deficiency and so replacement of the missing leptin should correct this problem, just as insulin injections correct insulin deficiency or diabetes. Leptin also produces a small amount of weight loss in normal mice. A very rare syndrome of leptin deficiency has just been found in two British children (see Chapter 3) but obese people generally have higher blood leptin levels than lean people. This may suggest a reduced response or insensitivity to leptin in obese people which would dampen enthusiasm about its potential for treating human obesity. In mice, sensitivity to leptin varies from complete unresponsiveness in one form of genetic obesity through to the high sensitivity of the ob/ob mouse, with normal lean mice somewhere between these two extremes. It is discouraging to note that mice made obese by feeding them a high fat diet, have high blood leptin levels and are less sensitive to injected leptin than normal mice.

Another problem with leptin is that it, like insulin, is a protein hormone and so it would also, like insulin, have to be given by injection rather than by mouth. Some very early trials of leptin injections in small numbers of obese people produced only slightly more weight loss over a three-month period than placebo injections.

Surgical treatment of obesity

Surgery is the last resort treatment for severe and intractable obesity. All surgical procedures carry some risk and this is much higher in obese people. Surgical treatment does seem to offer some help in losing weight to severely obese people and it may even be the most effective treatment for this extreme group judged purely on the basis of weight lost. Surgery is not an alternative to dieting, it is a way of helping patients to keep to their diets. Patients who overcome the barriers to excessive calorie intake that surgery introduces will not lose weight.

The most common procedure involves reducing the capacity of the stomach by surgically stapling off a large part of it. This means that the patient can only eat small meals; if they eat too much then this may cause them to vomit.

Jaw wiring involves wiring the jaws together so that the intake of solid food is restricted whereas the intake of liquids is relatively unhindered. This procedure is often effective in producing short-term weight loss whilst the jaws are actually wired, but patients usually regain the weight once the wires are removed. This wiring must be very socially restricting but the procedure may be useful for achieving short-term weight loss prior to surgery.

Conclusions

- Neither drugs nor surgery are really alternatives to diet and exercise, they simply aim to make it easier for patients to stick to their weight loss programme.
- Neither drugs nor surgery can be totally risk-free. Their use should therefore be restricted to cases where the benefits of their use are considered sufficient to outweigh these risks e.g. severe and intractable obesity.
- Although many compounds are being tested and evaluated as potential anti obesity drugs, there are currently very few drugs available and these are of limited effectiveness. This is particularly so since the recent withdrawl of fenfluramine and dexfenfluramine, two of the most effective and widely used drugs.

8 | POLITICS AND POLICY

Scope of the chapter

In these last few pages of the book, I have shifted the focus away from the individual reader and have taken a wider view to consider what can be done at the population/policy level to combat the rising tide of obesity in our countries. I have identified measures and resources that, as consumers and voters, we should be trying to extract from governments, and the food industry. I have also indicated, what, as parents, we can do to lessen the risk of our children becoming obese when they reach adulthood.

The population approach to reducing obesity

When treating obese individuals, the aim is substantial weight loss within a reasonable time. When dealing with population measures to reduce obesity prevalence then the benefits are expected to take years or decades to emerge rather than the weeks or months of an individual weight loss programme. When dealing with populations then one is seeking to arrest and eventually reverse the current year-on-year increases in the number of people who are overweight or obese. The odd decimal point off an individual's BMI is of limited significance but the same amount off the average population BMI would be significant – even preventing any further increases would be an achievement!

Obesity is already dreaded by the vast majority of the population, most overweight people would very much like to be thinner, many people fail to lose weight despite being desperate to succeed. Campaigns that aim to persuade people that being overweight or obese is undesirable and a detriment to their health are therefore pointless because that battle is already won. This victory has not, however, prevented obesity rates from spiralling ever upwards. Campaigns that focus upon the excess weight itself are therefore unlikely to produce benefits in terms of obesity reduction and may well just increase the unhappiness of overweight people and encourage even more denigration and discrimination. Rather, we must seek to identify and encourage changes in the behaviour of the whole population that favour better weight control. It is possible to produce major changes in a population's behaviour by persuasion and largely on health grounds. The dietary changes that Britons and Americans have been persuaded to make since the 1960s clearly demonstrates this. Over the past 30 years huge numbers have been persuaded to make the following health-related changes to their diets:

- To give up butter and replace it with soft polyunsaturated margarine and more recently with low fat spreads. Even in 1975, butter represented over two-thirds of the UK market for spreading fats and soft margarine just 14 per cent. By 1992, butter represented less than a quarter of this market with three-quarters going to soft margarine and the newer low fat spreads.
- To stop using lard and other animal fats for cooking and use vegetable oils instead. In 1975, lard accounted for about 70 per cent of sales of non-spreading fats in the UK and vegetable oils just 22 per cent. By 1992 these figures had almost exactly reversed.
- To replace much of the whole milk they consume with low fat milks.
- To replace much of the white bread they eat with bread made from less refined flour.
- To consume vast quantities of drinks sweetened with artificial sweeteners rather than sugar.

If we are to change population behaviour in ways that favour better weight control then we must do three things:

- identify and prioritise those changes in lifestyle and diet which would achieve better weight control with the least 'pain' to consumers;
- educate and motivate the population to make these changes;
- ensure that people have the opportunity and the means to make these changes.

What should the objectives be?

We must identify a small number of key objectives, make them clear priorities and concentrate our efforts on achieving them. I would suggest that two objectives should be given priority, namely:

- to increase the activity and fitness levels of our populations;
- to reduce the proportion of dietary calories that are derived from fat;

The reasons for choosing these particular priorities are discussed at length in Chapter 4. Both of these changes would lead to substantial improvements in health in their own right as well as favouring better weight control (see list on p.121). A reduction in dietary fat would inevitably also make the diet bulkier (i.e. lower its energy density) and would probably bring about other secondary changes in the diet that are considered desirable such as increased fibre intake. If a population is reasonably active and has a diet that has only moderate amounts of fat (ideally not more than 30 per cent of the calories compared to a current figure of close to 40 per cent) then this creates conditions where the natural energy balance control mechanisms are likely to be more effective when eating is not restrained. In the long-term, this should favour lower population levels of obesity.

You may wonder why I haven't included eating fewer calories and reducing sugar intake as specific objectives for the population. Recent rises in obesity prevalence seem to have occurred at a time when calorie intake has also been falling (see Chapter 4 Figure 4.1) and so just recommending people to eat even less food does not seem to be the way forward. If we focus upon sugar reduction and more sugar is replaced by artificial sweeteners, then these lost sugar calories may be partly replaced by fat which is poorly detected by our natural intake control mechanisms. In general people who eat low sugar diets tend to eat high fat diets (sugar-fat-seesaw) and these people are more likely to be overweight than people on high sugar, low fat diets.

Education and publicity

Education starts with the young and with schools. Schools could do much more to encourage *all* of their pupils to be physically active and to teach their pupils about diet, food composition and the skills of food preparation. Prevention of obesity by changing the lifestyle of the young will be easier than trying to treat established obesity in adults.

Physical education in schools

In many schools, certainly in the UK, physical education is not given a high enough priority – it may be seen as taking time away from the 'more important' academic subjects. Sometimes the priority of games teaching, and especially extra-curricular sessions, seems to be to develop the talents of the gifted and enthusiastic minority and so to produce winners who will enhance the school's prestige. There is often overemphasis on team games and sports that are difficult to continue playing into adulthood. Physical education must be made as inclusive as possible. People of all abilities and aptitudes must be given every opportunity to participate, to *enjoy* their participation and to develop their skills and talents no matter how limited they may be. There must be more attention given to developing skills and interests in active pursuits that are easier to continue in adult life. Developing natural talent and allowing participation in team games are excellent aims provided they are not done to the exclusion of all else. How would we feel about a school which was excellent at developing its academically gifted pupils but left many of the rest illiterate and innumerate? How would we feel about a school whose curriculum concentrated almost exclusively upon developing knowledge and skills that would be largely unused in adult life?

How parents can help

Of course, making children more active involves more than just increasing participation in gym lessons and formal games. It is also about encouraging them to be more active in their free time and incorporating more 'necessary' activity into their daily schedule. Parents must play a major part here by encouraging their children to walk and cycle rather than ride everywhere, by encouraging them to be more active in their leisure time and perhaps by encouraging them to participate in active household and garden chores. Simply reducing the amount of time spent watching TV or playing computer games is likely to increase a child's activity. These may keep them contented or at least quiet but their overuse is not in the child's best interest. Parents need to be persuaded that plenty of physical activity is necessary for growing children just as they accept the necessity for good food. They need to be made aware of just how inactive their children currently are. Many of us would be shocked at the results if we kept a log of how much time our children spend in front of a TV or computer screen during a week. Active parents and teachers are good role models for encouraging children to be active.

Health promotion for all

In health promotion messages aimed at the whole population then we must suggest realistic strategies for increasing activity and suggest realistic targets. We must, of course, encourage people to participate in active leisure time pursuits but we must also try to get people to incorporate more activity into their everyday schedule. There is currently a national advertising campaign in the UK aimed at encouraging people to take a thirty minute walk on most days. People must be convinced that exercise matters and will offer real benefits and they must also be made aware of just how inactive they are. The same surveys that have highlighted the extreme inactivity of British adults have also found high levels of complacency – many people consider that they are already reasonably fit and active. Perhaps they mistake being busy for being active.

Nutrition education

Food and nutrition, including food preparation skills, should be given proper weighting in the school curriculum. If people are to be encouraged to reduce their fat consumption, for instance, they must know where their dietary fat comes from and be clear about how to implement this advice. Many people, for example, do not know that ordinary soft margarine contains as much fat and as many calories as butter, and that vegetable oils are pure fat.

Adults as well as children need to be better educated about food composition and especially the sources of fat in their diets. They need to be offered simple, realistic and relatively painless ways of achieving the desired reduction in fat intake. I listed earlier some of the quite spectacular dietary changes that Britons and Americans have made over the last 30 years. Note that all of these changes involved the simple replacement of one product with another similar product and so they were easy to understand and implement. Even though the new healthier product is often considered slightly less palatable than the traditional one, people are prepared, in large numbers, to make this relatively small sacrifice. Table 6.3 lists a number of dietary modifications to 'save' fat.

Barriers to change

Why has the western world become so inactive? A large part of the answer is because technology has given us the freedom to choose, to be less active. We can drive rather than walk, we can replace human power with machine power in many home, garden and occupational tasks. Technology also offers us non-physical ways of pleasurably occupying our increased leisure time. There is not much that anyone can do about this – one probably cannot and should not attempt to legislate to restrict car usage, limit TV output or prevent the development of still more labour-saving devices on purely health grounds. There may well, however, be a case upon other grounds (the environment) for taking more active measures to discourage car usage. All that health educators can do is to seek to persuade people to use their cars and labour-saving devices more selectively and to occupy more of their leisure time with active pursuits.

It is also clear, however, that social, economic and environmental factors may act as barriers to discourage activity. People may sometimes feel forced to drive themselves or their children because of fears for their safety when walking or cycling:

- they may feel vulnerable as pedestrians or cyclists to accidental injury by motor vehicles;
- they may fear being mugged or their children being molested;
- the noise and pollution caused by motor vehicles may make walking or cycling unpleasant.

I am not going to try to suggest detailed solutions to these problems, I am not qualified to do so. However, I am suggesting that the safety and comfort of pedestrians and cyclists needs to be moved much higher up the political agenda. Politicians, town planners, law enforcement agencies and transport policy makers must seek ways of giving back the 'freedom of the streets' to non-car users. Some of these fears may be exaggerated or unfounded, in which case hard evidence needs to be produced and conveyed to the general public.

If people are to be encouraged to use their leisure time more actively then they must have easy and free access to attractive open areas. They must have easy and affordable access to sports and games facilities and these must be open at times when working people are able to make use of them. Obesity and inactivity are particularly prevalent amongst the lower socioeconomic groups and so privately built and commercially run facilities will probably charge fees that are beyond their means. National and local government will therefore have to play a major role in ensuring that such affordable facilities are available to all. Many employers also provide such facilities for their employees and more could be encouraged to do so, they might even be encouraged to provide 'opportunities' for activity in the working days of their employees. Could more use be made of school and college facilities outside normal school hours?

Why do we eat such a high fat diet?

As with inactivity, this is largely a matter of personal choice; we eat high fat food because we like it and can afford it. However, as we have seen earlier, people are prepared, in large numbers, to make dietary changes for the sake of their health. Are there any barriers that prevent people adopting a lower fat diet? Ignorance about the sources of fat in the diet and about ways of reducing the fat content is clearly one barrier which needs to be addressed through education and publicity. The range of low and reduced fat foods in the supermarket is enormous and growing rapidly – the food industry has been quick to recognise and supply this market. Although competitive pressures should ensure that supermarkets supply any public demands for healthier or low fat products, the profit motive may also not unreasonably encourage them to make special efforts with expensive specialist products and processed foods – so-called value added foods. This might disadvantage the poorer sections of the community. Supermarkets are also increasingly taking on a nutrition education and awareness role. They provide leaflets and posters on aspects of diet and health and information about food composition. Many supermarkets provide symbols on their products to indicate that foods are, for example, low in fat or salt or high in fibre or a particular nutrient. Provided this information is honest and reliable then this is a very positive development. The quality of this information needs to be monitored by consumer groups and regulatory authorities.

Examples of low or reduced fat foods now available in supermarkets:

- extra lean meat and poultry
- skimmed milk (essentially fat-free)
- low fat yoghurts
- reduced fat cheddar-type cheeses
- low fat cottage cheese
- reduced fat mayonnaise, and fat-free salad dressings
- low fat margarine-type spreads
- low fat cakes and biscuits (cookies)
- fish canned in water or brine rather than oil
- reduced fat French fries
- reduced fat potato crisps (chips) and other savoury snacks
- reduced/low fat ready meals.

Note that although these products contain less fat than the standard product some still contain substantial amounts of fat and so must still be used cautiously when trying to lose weight, for example, reduced fat cheddar cheese, low fat spreads and potato crisps (chips), some reduced fat ready meals. Some low fat products do contain substantial amounts of sugar, for example, many low fat yoghurts. Those unable to reach the large supermarkets may not have such ready access to these low fat options, small local shops and especially those in rural areas will probably stock a very restricted range of foods, especially perishable foods like fresh fruits and vegetables. Some caterers have also been relatively slow to incorporate low fat options into their menus. In many cafeterias in schools and factories, fast food outlets, restaurants etc low fat options are less apparent than on the supermarket shelf.

It is often said that eating a healthy, low fat diet should make eating cheaper. This may be true if some expensive foods from the meat and milk groups and some fatty prepared foods are replaced by more bread, potatoes and inexpensive vegetables. However, this is an unappealing option for most people; they want to be healthier but without radically restructuring their diet and with minimum loss of palatability. They want to eat more of the most desirable fruits and vegetables and to replace high fat foods with lower fat versions, for example, leaner meat, low fat milk, low fat spreads and low fat versions of prepared foods. Such changes do involve increased costs and may limit the ability of poorer people to change. If one is trying to provide enough calories for a family with limited money, then foods high in fat and sugar often provide lots of calories per penny – lower fat versions usually provide many fewer calories per penny and most fruits and vegetables are very poor buys using 'calories per penny' as the criterion. Perhaps this is one more reason why obesity is more prevalent in the lower socioeconomic groups.

Conclusions

- Tackling the problem of obesity at the population level requires a long-term co-ordinated strategy designed to slow down, arrest and eventually reverse the current upward trends in average BMI and obesity rates.
- These strategies must concentrate on promoting and facilitating desirable behaviour change rather than focusing upon the dangers of overweight and obesity. There is already an almost universal desire to remain or become lean.
- Increasing physical activity and reducing fat consumption are identified as the priority aims for reducing population rates of obesity.
- Encouragement and education are obviously important in increasing activity and moderating fat consumption. However, we must also identify and tackle the barriers that prevent many people being more active and eating less fat.
- Increased participation in leisure-time activity is an important goal. However, we must also find ways of making our streets safer and more convenient for walkers and cyclists so that people can incorporate more activity into their everyday schedules.

GLOSSARY

Adaptive thermogenesis an increase in heat production – the function of which is to burn off surplus calories and prevent excessive weight gain. Suggested to occur in **brown fat**.

Amphetamine one of the first anti-obesity drugs. It works by increasing the actions of the **nerve transmitter noradrenaline (norepinephrine)**. It also increases the actions of another nerve transmitter called dopamine and this produces a potentially addictive euphoric effect. Amphetamine derivatives have been produced in which this dopamine effect is minimised. The effectiveness of these drugs is only temporary.

Anorexia Nervosa a potentially fatal **eating disorder** which is characterised by an obsessive desire to be thin and self-starvation.

Appestat centres in the brain which monitor body energy stores and control feeding to prevent over- or under-feeding. Analogous to a thermostat controlling temperature.

Appetite the hedonistic desire to eat c.f. **hunger**.

Aerobic using oxygen. Thus **aerobic exercise** is moderate exercise where the oxygen supply to the muscles is sufficient to allow it to generate the required energy by normal aerobic means. **Aerobic capacity** is a scientific measure of fitness – the capacity of the heart and lungs to deliver oxygen to the muscles.

Anaerobic not using oxygen. Thus **anaerobic exercise** is intense exercise where the supply of oxygen is insufficient to generate all of the required energy and so some is generated by other non-oxygen-requiring methods (e.g. weight lifting).

Basal Metabolic Rate, (BMR) the rate of energy expenditure (metabolic rate) in the resting or basal state i.e. lying down, in a warm room and some time after eating. The minimum metabolic rate in a conscious person.

ß₃-adrenoreceptor a receptor found specifically on **brown fat cells**. Drugs that stimulate this receptor should increase heat production and burn off surplus calories.

ß-carotene a substance found in many green and brightly coloured fruits and vegetables which acts as a source of vitamin A.

Behaviour therapy a psychological approach to the treatment of obesity. Subjects modify their behaviour to avoid situations that trigger inappropriate eating behaviour and reward appropriate behaviours e.g. taking exercise.

Body Mass Index, (BMI) the weight in kilogrammes divided by the height in metres squared. A BMI of under 20 is classified as underweight, 25–30 is classified as **overweight** and a BMI of over 30 as **obese**.

Brown fat literally fat tissue that is brown. Is prominent in small mammals, hibernators and human babies and is known to be capable of generating considerable amounts of heat. Could be the site at which surplus calories are burnt off (**adaptive thermogenesis**).

Bulimia Nervosa an **eating disorder** characterised by bouts of gorging followed by induced vomiting, fasting, frenetic exercise or laxative use. Sufferers may have a normal body weight.

Butabindide a chemical that protects **cholecystokinin** from breakdown in the brain and so increases its effects. May have potential as an appetite suppressant drug.

Cafeteria feeding a method of increasing fatness in lab animals by allowing them access to a variety of tasty and fattening foods. Regarded as the best animal model of human obesity.

Calorie a common unit of energy in nutrition. When used by nutritionists and in this book it strictly means a thousand calories (a kilocalorie).

Carbohydrate-fat seesaw the observation that as the proportion of energy from carbohydrate goes up so that from fat tends to go down and vice versa. Similarly there also appears to be a sugar- fat seesaw – high proportion of calories from sugar relatively low proportion from fat. As high fibre diets tend to be low in fat and vice versa one might also argue that there tends to be a fibre-fat seesaw.

Catastrophising   exaggerating the effects of a small lapse in a diet e.g. saying that a chocolate bar has undone the benefits of weeks of successful dieting.

Cholecystokinin, (CCK)   a hormone released from the gut after feeding that stimulates bile production. It may also act as a **satiety signal** by stimulating sensing nerves in the gut. CCK is also found in the brain where it acts as a **nerve transmitter**.

db/db (*diabetes*) **mouse**   a genetic form of obesity in mice. These mice appear to be unable to respond to **leptin**.

Dexfenfluramine   as **fenfluramine**.

Dietary fibre   indigestible material (largely carbohydrate) found only in plant foods. Found in greatest amounts in unrefined plant foods, e.g. whole grain cereals, whole fruits and vegetables (especially unpeeled).

Energy balance   the difference between the energy taken in as food and drink and that expended by the body. A zero balance would imply weight stability in adults. A positive energy balance indicates that there is growth of lean tissue or increased fat storage whereas a negative energy balance implies loss of fat and/or lean.

High Density Lipoproteins, (HDL)   fat and protein complexes in the blood that contain cholesterol. They protect against heart disease and so are referred to as the 'good cholesterol'.

5-HT(serotonin)   a **nerve transmitter** in the brain that is involved in feeding control. Substances that increase the action of 5-HT in the brain suppress appetite, e.g. **fenfluramine** and **dexfenfluramine**.

Hypothalamus   a part of the brain, the location of the **appestat**. Damage to the ventromedial hypothalamus leads to overeating and obesity in animals whereas damage to the lateral hypothalamus abolishes eating behaviour. The notion that these two areas contained centres that control all eating behaviour is called the dual-centre hypothalamus but is now considered too simplistic.

Eating disorder   a general term that includes **anorexia nervosa**, **bulimia nervosa** and people whose eating behaviour is abnormal but falls shorts of the diagnostic criteria for these diseases.

Energy density   the energy concentration of a food or diet. The number of calories in a given weight. Fatty foods have very high energy density whereas foods with high water content (e.g. most fruits and leafy vegetables) have low energy density.

Fenfluramine   a widely used appetite suppressant drug that acts by increasing the actions of the **nerve transmitter** known as **5-HT (serotonin)**. At the time of writing this drug has been withdrawn by the manufacturers after a report of possible side-effects.

Food combining   a dietary system formulated by an American physician, William Hay. The distinctive feature is that high protein and high carbohydrate foods should not be eaten together. The scientific basis of this is regarded as false by nutritionists.

Glucostat theory   the notion that blood glucose concentration is a major factor controlling feeding. High blood glucose causes satiation but low blood glucose causes hunger.

Glycogen   animal form of starch, stored in relatively small amounts in liver and muscle of non-fasting people.

Hunger   the physiological drive or need to eat c.f. **appetite**.

Insulin   a hormone produced in the pancreas which controls blood glucose concentration. Lack of insulin is the cause of diabetes.

Ketones   substances produced in the liver from fat during prolonged fasting. They are used as an energy source by the brain. Produced in excess in severe, untreated diabetes. Impart an 'alcohol' or 'pear drops' smell to the breath.

Ketosis   having high concentrations of ketones in the blood, e.g. mildly during starvation or carbohydrate deprivation or severely in some untreated diabetics.

Kilojoule   a unit of energy. One **calorie** (strictly one kilocalorie) is equal to 4.2 kilojoules.

Leptin   a newly discovered hormone produced in fat tissue. Its concentration in blood seems to reflect and thus indicate to the **appestat** the size of the body fat stores. May have potential for obesity treatment.

Lipase   the enzyme that digests fat in the gut. Produced in the pancreas.

Lipostat theory   the notion that the **appestat** can detect the size of body fat stores and control feeding to maintain these stores at a fixed level (see **leptin**).

Nerve transmitters   chemical substances which nerves use to 'communicate', they are released from nerves and they activate or inhibit other nerves, muscles or glands.

Neuropeptide Y   a key **nerve transmitter** in the brain in the control of feeding. Injecting it into the brains of animals increases feeding.

Non Insulin dependent diabetes Mellitus, (NIDDM)   the relatively mild form of diabetes that starts in later life. Strongly associated with obesity, NIDDM predisposes to heart disease, kidney disease, blindness and gangrene.

Noradrenaline (norepinephrine)   a **nerve transmitter** involved in control of feeding. **Amphetamines** increase the actions of noradrenaline and so suppress appetite.

ob/ob (obese) mouse   a genetically obese mouse widely used in obesity research. The obesity appears to be due to a defect in the gene for **leptin**.

Obese   a **Body Mass Index** of over 30.

Oedema (US edema)   swelling of tissues due to excess water content. A symptom of several diseases, local injury and of severe malnutrition.

Olestra   an artificial fat which cannot be digested. If added to food it gives some of the palatability effects of fat without adding calories.

Orlistat   a drug that blocks fat digestion and so reduces its absorption from the gut.

Overweight   a **Body Mass Index**, in the range 25-30.

Placebo   a dummy drug or treatment.

Physical Activity Level, (PAL)   When estimating energy expenditure, the number by which the **Basal Metabolic Rate** is multiplied to allow for energy used in the day's activity. Ranges from around 1.3 (e.g. housebound elderly person) to well over 2 (e.g. a serious athlete in training).

Rebound hypoglycaemia   a fall in blood glucose to below the starting level within a short time of eating which produces hunger. Associated with refined and rapidly digested foods.

Retinol   vitamin A.

Risk factors   factors such as high blood pressure, high blood cholesterol and obesity, that predict a higher risk of developing a particular disease.

Satiety signals   physiological signals that indicate to the **appestat** the feeding state and level of body energy stores. They produce satiation, and their absence leads to **hunger**.

Sensory specific satiety   describes the phenomenon whereby, during eating ones, appetite for a previously consumed food diminishes rapidly but one's appetite for other foods is much less affected. As a consequence, increased variety might favour overeating.

Set point   refers to the notion that body weight control mechanisms operate to maintain a fixed level of body–fatness analogous to a thermostat set to maintain a fixed temperature.

Sibutramine   a potential anti-obesity drug. It acts to increase the actions of both **5-HT (serotonin)** and **noradrenaline (norepinephrine)** in the brain.

State registered dietitian, (SRD) a formal and recognised dietetics qualification in the UK.

Thermogenic   produces heat, e.g. a thermogenic drug stimulates heat production and could burn off surplus calories.

Very low calorie diets, (VLCDs)   diets designed to contain only a few hundred calories but all of the essential nutrients, usually taken in the form of meal replacement drinks.

Waist-to-hip ratio   the ratio of body circumference around the waist to that at the hips. A high ratio (apple shape) indicates a predominance of abdominal fat, a low ratio (pear shape) a predominance of fat on the hips and under the skin. A high ratio makes being **overweight** or **obese** more hazardous.

'Yo-yo' dieting   cycles of weight loss and regain.

FURTHER READING

Doyle, W, 1994. *Teach Yourself Healthy Eating*. London: Hodder and Stoughton.

Gibbs, W W, 1996. 'Gaining on fat'. *Scientific American,* August 1996 issue, p.70–76.

Pool, R, 1997. 'Things can only get worse'. *New Scientist,* 23 August 1997 issue p.22–27.

Prentice, A M and Jebb, S A, 1995. 'Obesity in Britain: gluttony or sloth?' *British Medical Journal* **311**, 437–439 (12 August 1995 issue).

Rink, T J, 1994. 'In search of a satiety factor'. *Nature* **372**, 406–407.

Sizer, F S and Whitney, E N, 1994. *Nutrition. Concepts and controversies.* 6th edn. St. Paul, MN: West Publishing Company.

Webb, G P, 1995. *Nutrition: a health promotion approach.* London: Arnold.

Webb, G P and Copeman, J, 1996. *The nutrition of older adults.* London: Arnold.

INDEX

USEFUL ADDRESSES

Family physicians may be able to recommend counsellors specialising in particular sorts of therapies or local self-help groups. Telephone directories may also contain lists of counsellors, dietitians, sports' centres, fitness clubs, local slimming clubs and local Weight Watchers branches. Local health promotion units, often attached to local hospitals, may also be useful sources of both direct help and guidance towards others who can provide appropriate help or guidance.

United Kingdom

Anorexia Aid
The Priory Centre
11 Priory Road
High Wycombe
Bucks
tel. 01494-21431

British Dietetic Association
Elizabeth House
Suffolk Street
Birmingham B1 1LS
tel. 0121-643 5483
Web Page: http://www.bda.uk.com

Food and Drink Federation
(The FDF Campaign for Physical
Activity and Health Eating)
6 Catherine Street
London WC2B 5JJ
tel. 0171-836 2460
Obesity Lifeline tel. 0181-203 3441

British Diabetic Association
10 Queen Anne Street
London W1M 0BD
tel. 0171-253 3406

Eating Disorders Association
Sackville Place
44 Magdalen Street
Norwich
Norfolk NR3 1JU
tel. 01603-621414

Health Education Authority
Hamilton House
Mabledon Place
London WC1H 9TX
tel. 0171-413 2637

Obesity Resource Information
Centre (ORIC)
40-42 Osnaburgh Street
London NW1 3ND
tel. 0171-465 0130

Slimmer Clubs UK
Unit 4
Cholswell Court
Cholswell Road
Abingdon
Oxon OX13 6HW
tel. 01235-550700

Sports Nutrition Foundation
London Sports Medicine Institute
c/o Medical College
St Bartholomew's Hospital
Charterhouse Square
London EC1M 6BQ
tel. 0171-251 0583

Weight Watchers (UK) LTD.
Kidwells Park Road
Maidenhead
Berkshire SL6 8BP
tel. 0345-123000

Scottish Health Education Group
Woodburn House
Canaan Lane
Edinburgh EH10 4SG
tel. 0131-536 5500

The Sport's Council
16 Upper Woburn Place
London WC1 8QP
tel. 0171-273 1500

The Vegetarian Society
Parkdale
Dunham Road
Altrincham
Cheshire WA14 4QG
tel. 0161-928 0793

Women's Nutritional
Advisory Service
P.O. Box 268
Lewes
East Sussex BN7 2QN
tel. 01273-467366

United States

American Anorexia and Bulimia
Association, Inc.
418 East 76th Street
New York, NY 10021
tel. (212) 734-1114

American Diabetes Association
660 Duke Street

American Dietetic
Association (ADA)
216 West Jackson Boulevard,
Suite 800
Chicago, IL 60606-6995
tel. (312) 899-0040
Anorexia Nervosa and Related
Eating Disorders (ANRED)

Alexandria, VA 22314
tel. (703) 549-1500
tel. (800) 232-3472

Bulimia Anorexia Self-Help
Crisis Line
tel. (800) 227-4785
tel. (800) 762-3347

Consumer's Union
101 Truman Avenue
Yonkers, NY 10703-1057
tel. (914) 378-2000

FDA Office of Nutrition and
Food Sciences
200 C Street SW
Washington, DC 20204
tel. (202) 205-4561

National Association of Anorexia
Nervosa and Associated Disorders,
Inc. (ANAD)
P.O. Box 7
Highland Park, IL. 60035
tel. (708) 831-3438

National Council Against Health
Fraud Inc.
P.O. Box 1276
Loma Linda, CA 92354

Overeaters Anonymous (OA)
383 Van Ness Avenue, Suite 1601

P.O. Box 5102
Eugene, OR 97405
tel. (503) 344-1114

Consumer Information Center
Department 609K
Pueblo, CO 81009

Food and Drug Administration
(FDA)
Office of Consumer Affairs
HFE 881 Room 16-63
5600 Fishers Lane
Rockville MD 20857
Consumer Information Line
tel. (301) 443-3170

Grace-Full Eating (Fat acceptance
newsletter)
Terry Garrison
Annabel Taylor Hall
Cornell University
Ithaca, NY 14853

National Association to Advance
Fat Acceptance (NAAFA)
P.O. Box 188620
Sacramento, CA 95818
tel. (916) 558-6880

USDA Human Nutrition
Information Service
6505 Belcrest Road
Federal Building One,
Room 325-A
Hyattsville, MD 20782
tel. (202) 720-2791
T.O.P.S. (Take Off Pounds
Sensibly)

Torrace, CA 90501

P.O. Box 07360
Milwaukee, WI 53207

U.S. Department of Education (DOE)
Accreditation Agency Evaluation
Branch
7th and D Street SW
Building 3, Room 336
Washington, DC 20202
tel. (202) 708-7417

Weight Watchers
Consumer Affairs Department A
500 North Broadway
Jericho, NY 11753-2196
tel. (800) 874-4170

Canada

Canadian Diabetes Association
15 Toronto Street, Suite 1001
Toronto
Ontario M5G 2E3

Canadian Dietetic Association
480 University Avenue, Suite 604
Toronto
Ontario M5G 1V2
tel. (416) 596-0857

Consumers' Association of Canada
307 Gilmour Street
Ottawa
Ontario K2P 0P7

National Eating Disorders
Information Centre
200 Elizabeth Street,
College Wing 1-328
Toronto
Ontario M5G 2C4

Nutrition Programs Unit
Health Promotion Directorate
Health Canada
4th Floor, Jeanne Mance Building
Tunney's Pasture
Ottawa
Ontario K1A 0L3

Other countries

Association for Dietetics
in South Africa
P.O. Box 4309
Randburg 2125
tel. 11 886 8130

Irish Nutrition and Dietetic Institute
Ashgrove House
Kill Avenue
Dun Laoghaire
Co Dublin
tel. 01-2804 839

Weight Watchers (Australia)
5th Floor
40 Miller Street
North Sydney 2060
New South Wales
tel. 011-612-9928 1300

Weight Watchers (South Africa)
11th Floor
Corner Bertha
Jorssen Street
Bloomfontein
tel. 5127 1133 93527

Dietitians Association of Australia
1/8 Phipps Close
Deakin ACT 2600
tel. 2 6282 0555
Web Page: http://www.daa.asn.au

The New Zealand Dietetic
Association
P.O. Box 5065
Wellington
tel. 4 472 7421

Weight Watchers (New Zealand)
P.O. Box 1328
Auckland
tel. 0116-4936-02345

INVESTIGATING PSYCHOLOGY:
A PRACTICAL APPROACH FOR NURSING

Lesley A. Wattley, BA, SRN
Lecturer in Nursing Studies
Welsh National School of Medicine
Cardiff

Dave J. Müller, PhD, BEd, ABPsS
Senior Lecturer in Psychology
South Glamorgan Institute of Higher Education
Cardiff

Foreword by
Christine Chapman, BSc, MPhil, SRN, SCM, RNT, FRCN,
Director of Nursing Studies
Welsh National School of Medicine

Harper & Row, Publishers
London

Cambridge		San Francisco
Hagerstown		Mexico City
Philadelphia		São Paulo
New York		Sydney

First published 1984
Reprinted 1985

Harper & Row Ltd
28 Tavistock Street
London WC2E 7PN

British Library Cataloguing in Publication Data
Wattley, Lesley
    Investigating psychology.
    1. Nursing—Psychological aspects
    I. Title   II. Müller, Dave
    150'.24613   RT86
    ISBN 0-06-318261-0

Typeset by BookEns, Saffron Walden
Printed and bound in Great Britain by
Butler & Tanner Ltd, Frome and London